Fascia

How Decompressing Your Fascia is the Missing Link in Healing

(Work Your Fascia to Free Your Body Relieve Pain, Boost Your Energy, Ease Anxiety and Depression)

Steven Jones

Published By **Darby Connor**

Steven Jones

Fascia: How Decompressing Your Fascia is the Missing Link in Healing (Work Your Fascia to Free Your Body Relieve Pain, Boost Your Energy, Ease Anxiety and Depression)

ISBN   978-1-7776534-7-7

Legal & Disclaimer

Table Of Contents

Chapter 1: Network Fasciae

Why fasciae from every kind are affect your health? What do they have to offer in the first place?

To answer the questions above, let's begin with a brief explanation of the word. The word "fascia" is derived from Latin which is a reference to a bundle. If fasciae (Greek mys) and fascia create one unit that is inseparable that is also known as myofascia. It's now recognized by scientists that the sensorium of fasciae plays a major importance to a well-being and well-being body. Fasciae also play a role in an extent for shaping (morphology) of the body. The network of various types of connective tissue is a part of all of our body. Therefore, it connects the various body parts effectively and holistically with each with each.

There are six primary functional myo-fascial links within the body.

The dorsal line that runs across the surface extends from below the foot up to the eyebrows. The main characteristic of this line is that it withstands the pressure and maintains the posture of an upright person and also acts as a stifle (counterpart) in opposition to the frontal line that is superficial.

The line that runs along the frontal surface runs from the upper part of the feet to side of skull. It's anatomically split in two sections, however practically speaking, it must be considered as one unit, because there is no continuous link between the upper and legs. In general, it offers fast strength and protects your posture and actions as well as acts as a antagonist (counterpart) for the surface back line.

A deep line of frontal symmetry runs beginning from the inner side of the feet to the sides of your legs (adductors) the pelvis and the spine's front and chest up to the external side of the skull. It is a characteristically functional and stabilizing connection within the body.

The lateral line runs that runs from your ankles' outsides towards the ear. The main reason for this is it helps to maintain stability and balance to your body's position and posture.

The spiral line begins and ends in the occiput. It follows the shoulder opposite, crossing over the top of the body near the diaphragm's level and runs along the outer side of the leg until the inner side of the feet. It continues to expands across the arches of your foot, extending along the sacrum, and then the dorsal extensor towards the Occipital. Its uniqueness is that it gives stability, flexibility, and the ability to balance.

Four arm lines provide maximal mobility while maintaining stability. They comprise:

The frontal arm's superficial line. It starts at the smaller side of your chest, and traverses the clavicles, middle ribs, the small pectorals, the large back muscles, the thoracic spine before ending at the pelvis.

The lower-lying arm line. It starts at the pectoral muscle of the small and continues through the radius, arm wrist and finally with the ball of thumb.

The posterior extremity of the superficial line. It is located from the back of the skull and is above the 12th vertebra, and then across the shoulder's front and across the arm extensor, and behind of the hand, and finally to the fingers.

The deeper posterior arm line. It starts at the spinous processes in the thoracic upper and lower cervical spines and extends across shoulder blades until the flexor arm of the upper arm.

It's remarkable how this connective tissue connects to each other and, in doing so, facilitates and can influence, for example the coordination between different muscles chains. The more frequently our fasciae get cared for and maintained, the better they influence the performance of our bodies and sensation.

The more vigorous we lead our life, the more beneficially our fasciae develop as well as the bones and muscles. The more restless our lives become, the greater infected the connective tissue becomes and the more weak and less efficient the performance of our bodies.

In our daily lives throughout our lives, we develop both negative and positive movements through our everyday behaviors, that are then stored in our brains and are recalled at times of need. Fascia is a very similar brain that learns and consequently can impact our posture as well as our psyche. If we modify our routines and habits, and are more active adverse reactions as well as bad" motion patterns could be corrected. Therefore, we can have an impact on the perception of our body of posture, reactions and regularly moving the fasciae.

The effects of facial disorders are severe and can alter the functioning of the human system" and can cause among others extreme pain, nausea, and even feelings of general apprehension.

Chapter 2: Cause Of Pain Fasciae

What causes pain? It is experienced in our brain. It is also experienced it. There are various pain receptors all over the tissues of our body. Alpha-delta fibers play a role in the sense of an abrupt sensation of pain. The feeling of pain that is picked up through these fibers and relayed to our brains via neural pathways that guide nerves, generally is sudden and abruptly. A good example of this would be when we rub our shin unintentionally. The majority of the time, it takes just about a few seconds for us to experience the pain as being sharp extremely intense and abrupt (in our brains). In contrast it is a possibility that we've hurt yourself a time long ago, and are left with the bruising, i.e. an insignificant hematoma from the accident, or experience muscular soreness or tension or from a vigorous training of the muscles, or from an unintentional physical exercise, the C-fibers transmit a dull low" sensation for the brain.

It is typically an uncomfortable, however manageable discomfort.

The various forms of perception are based on the same thing that they all share: they influence our life. For instance, by using an appropriate posture or even not moving, which is essential for healthy, well-maintained fasciae as well as for well-being.

A different type of pain, that is common for the majority of people it is usually felt as being in the back. It is among the leading causes of incapacitation for work, and is the third most frequent reason for visiting the doctor. Naturally, it can cause profound social and psychosomatic consequences for those who are who are affected. The latest research shows that the signal of pain emanating from the back may be traced to the posterior lumbar ligament in the lower back.

Because the fasciae contain many sensors, in the case of a growing hardening, thickening or even tearing of these structures, signals for pain instantly get sent to the brain by the central and peripheral nerve pathways for guidance. This means that we know something is not right and may also send an immediate feedback to the signal sender and the conductor, called the fascia. The body can respond to the signals for pain from the fascia by caring for precisely this organ of sensory stimulation within our bodies frequently and addressing it with specificity. So back pain can be cured in short time. It's all it takes is some discipline, determination and routine.

The benefits of strong fascia tissues are apparent, since regular treatment of the fascia can resolve persistent and often chronic difficulties. Connective tissue that is healthy has an empowering, protecting as well as a stabilizing properties. It could even assist your immune system fight off illnesses.

TREAT FASCIA REGULARLY

Self-care that is consistent and focused of your fasciae will stimulate the tension system of your fasciae. Your investment in this will be a great reward for the client! If the fascial system of your body is in good working order, any problems can be resolved swiftly. It can also have an immediate impact on our muscles. If both structures of fascia and muscle are healthy, flexible and well-positioned, we'll feel more youthful and healthier. In the same time it will provide safeguards against muscle injuries. You will be able to move as smooth like the cat". Here are a few excellent reasons for why frequent self-treatment of your fasciae could be beneficial.

Benefits of regular self-treatment include that routinely moving(s) or stressing(s) connective tissues (fascia) could help to protect the health of your body, avoid myofascial adhesions and instabilities and help maintain mobility through older aged. Simple tasks like packing shopping bags, carrying out household chores or climbing stairs should eventually be no problem for the person who is.

If your fascial system is healthy and well-maintained it is easier to stay fit and can boost your immunity and are able to live daily life, without worry and, above all, pain-free or less painful due to improved mobility. Its added value easily observable and noticeable whenever you go out with your friends on outdoor activities, and so you are doing something for your self. Your body and soul will be grateful.

Chapter 3: Exercise Collection At A Glance

If you want to be successful in tackling the task or undertaking, you must follow the rule of"Plan to Do Plan - Do Check Do - Act". Only people who are conscious of their goals, have developed the concept, and taken a vow to an level, will be able to execute effectively.

You will not only take a giant step closer towards your dream of a well-maintained fascia, but you can achieve it when you take care of yourself

1. regularly,

2. varied,

3. motivating,

4. static,

5. active and with

6. Push and pull components.

The programs below for self-care of your fascia-related structures have been designed based on the concepts previously mentioned. By using these 10 programs, you will be able to transform your fasciae to form in a variety of as well as specific to your topic and create the basis to lead a more active and healthy life.

All programs will require just seven minutes per program. Be sure to have two or three square feet of free space surrounding your. In the next pages of the book, you'll discover both video- and written directions on how to complete every exercise. At first the most important thing is to complete the exercises in a slower pace and to do them in a controlled way. It is the same for any workout you do in the first time. In the future, you may accelerate your exercises slightly, however you need to complete them properly and with greater repetitions.

We'd be happy to provide a short description of the types of is on the table for you in terms of exercises and programs.

01 BASIC PROGRAM

1. Upper body bends

2. Stretching the upper back

3. Apple picking

4. Upper body tilt

5. Upper Body rotation

6. Arm swing

02 STRONG BACK

1. The upper body is bent when rotating.

2. Lower body bends as the upper part of it is bent.

3. Extension and flexion of the upper body.

4. The upper body bends by crossing legs

5. One Arm swing

6. Alternating upper body tilt

03 FIT BACK

1. The upper body is bent when you step. posture

2. Dog that is downward facing with heel step

3. Lunges and upper body stretch with the lunge

4. Arms fling

5. Leg fly

6. Dip the heel of your shoe

04 ELASTIC AS A FEATHER

1. Dog with a downward-facing face and hip rotation

2. Lateral arm swing

3. Leapfrog

4. Interspersed jumps across the line

5. Foot circles

6. Stand up and roll your toes

05 MOBILE SHOULDERS

1. Upper body tilt

2. Swing arm cross-legged

3. Wing swing

4. Cross under obstacle

5. Waxing

6. Lower leg circling

06 FLEXIBLE HIPS

1. Lateral lunges

2. Leg swings are crossed

3. A downward-looking dog that has Spine rotation

4. Forward bent arm swing in lunge

5. The upper body's side is bent while closed hands

6. Upper body bends in lunge

07 HIP, KNEE & FOOT

1. Dog looking down

2. Leg rollover

3. Alternating jumps

4. Double arm swing

5. Hurdle jumps

6. Spinning top

08 COORDINATION & MOBILITY

1. Skater

2. Apple picking

3. Upper body rotation

4. A leg swings across an obstacle

5. Balance of the standing

6. Lower leg circles

09 BODY FITNESS

1. The trunk bends and the heel kicks

2. Lunges and upper body stretch.

3. Tilt of the upper body with crossed legs

4. Arm is swung

5. Arm sling

6. Standing long jump

10 HEALTHY FASCIA

1. The upper part of the body bends when rotated

2. Alternating upper body bends

3. Leg flyer

4. Balancing

5. Diagonal crunch

6. Overstep

Chapter 4: Your 10 Fascia Programs

1. Upper back is bent.

Start with the most superficial back line. Set your feet about hip width between each other. The arms are hanging by the sides, next to your body. Keep your chin in your chest. Then, starting from this position inhale and gently bend your torso down one vertebra at an time. Be sure to stretch your fingertips to the maximum distance possible towards your feet. Try to reach around your legs using the hands of your feet, if you can. Your head should be lowered towards your knees so that your forehead lies on the kneecaps. If it is possible you can, the legs need to be stretched for the full time in the exercise. Inhale and then return to your starting place before resuming the exercise procedure.

Exercise 2: Upper body stretch

This exercise will increase the strength of your superficial frontal line. Inhale

Straighten your upper body and extend your arms up until your body creates a "Y". With this fluid motion You then extend your arms upwards. When you stretch be sure to keep the abdominal muscles to ensure that you're stable and safe until you are in the final place of the exercise. After exhaling, bring your hands to the initial place beside your body prior to continuing the motion.

It is possible to combine the first and second exercises, in alternating them. The exercises should be completed within a minute. If you are combining each exercise, do each one in turn for around two minutes. Try to get to the desired end point using slight movements that are springy to slowly expand the range of movement. It is important to complete these exercises in a safe and exact method. Two exercises are provided which focus on the two lateral lines.

Exercise 3 - Apple picking

Your arms should be raised vertically in a series of movements. Think of picking apples off a tree by using only just one hand. Do the "one-armed apple picking" in a series of steps, to ensure that both your left and right bodies lines must extend far. Once you've extended as high as you're able in your arms for approximately an hour, go back to your starting point by putting your arms back by your sides with your fingers pointed downwards towards the floor.

Exercise 4 - Tilt of the upper body

Lift your arms in alternating upwards. Move your hands as far as you can to either left and right depending on your preference, and diagonally upwards to the point that your head is tilted upwards. body to the side and extend your upwards the body line. Your eyes should remain straight in the direction of your eyes. Be sure that your feet are solidly planted on the ground. Do this repeatedly for approximately one minute.

Exercise 5 The upper body rotate

The goal of this exercise is getting the spiral line activated. From the beginning you're standing with your feet roughly hip-width apart. Your arms are hanging vertically parallel down. The arm should be bent 90 degrees, so that your forearm rests above or under your stomach and then put your hands to the side of your hip opposite. By inhaling, lift your other arm up by bending it as far back as is possible, in order to rotate your torso. Keep your eyes on the hand in which you are active. It is important to move your hips at a minimum. The arm that is not active continues to rest on the belly. After exhaling, move your active hand back to its starting point following the same route. Repeat this exercise for approximately one minute, before changing sides and doing the same exercise using the other hand.

Exercise 6 - Swing arm

Through this workout, you'll stimulate the lines of your arms. For this exercise, put your feet in a hip-width space and move your upper body forward approximately 45 to 45 degrees. Then, begin swinging your arms the same direction in front and behind your body, with as wide a flexibility as you can. Do this for approximately 1 minute. Be sure you perform the move in a smooth and unhurried manner without stopping.

It is best to create notes in your appointment immediately to make arrangements for the next facial treatment. Be aware that a 7-minute regularly investing in the body's health can dramatically improve the quality of your living!

Upper body is bent by rotating

Your feet should be hip-width between each other. The arms are hanging on your sides, close to your body. Keep your chin in your chest. Then, starting from this position and exhale, gradually bend your upper back to the side, vertebra after vertebra. Be sure to bring your fingertips in the direction you can towards the ground. Turn your body sidewards in this direction so you are able to look back in the direction of your foot. Keep this posture for a few seconds before returning to your original place. Repeat the movement with the opposite part of the body. Perform this movement with a steady and controlled movements for around 1 minute.

Upper lower body is bent in a lunge.

Stand in a tiny lunge, then put the sole of your front foot to the floor. The feet's toes face upwards. Your leg on the floor could be bent slightly. The front of your leg should be in a straight position. Keep your chin in your chest. Then, starting from this posture and exhale, gradually bend your upper back downwards, vertebra by vertebra. Grab the ankle of your forward foot with your fingers. Switch the legs. Repeat this workout for about 30 seconds on both sides.

Upper body is bent and stretched.

Your feet should be hip-width to each other. Your arms rest on your sides, close to your body. Put one of your legs backwards onto your feet and then raise the arms above your head. They should be parallel. Get yourself up. In this posture, you must simultaneously move your body forward and the back of your leg up by bringing your knee up to the forward bent torso. Your bent arms aid in the movement by swinging downwards and backwards. It takes around 1 minute.

Upper body tilt by crossing legs

Stand straight. Set your right foot behind the left one to ensure that the sides of your feet meet. Stand straight at the beginning during this workout by crossing your legs. Inhale and raise the right arm upwards vertically. Your left arm stays in the torso, and is hanging downwards vertically. Make sure to extend your left hand at least the left side diagonally over your head to notice a slight stretch to the right part of your body. Maintain this position for around 30 seconds. In this time and with a conscious exhalation attempt to move slightly higher to your left. Switch sides and feet postures and repeat this move with the opposite side for approximately half an hour and also.

Chapter 5: 5 One Arm Swings

Your feet should be hip-width to each other. The arms are between your legs in front of your body. Starting from this position move one arm between front as well behind you attentively watching the swing. Increase the intensity of your movement until you can swing your arm in the direction of as much forward and reverse as is possible. Do this for around one minute prior to changing sides and performing this exercise on the second arm. The entire exercise shouldn't take more than one minute on both arms.

Alternate the upper body tilt

Your body is upright and your feet firmly in touch. Your arms rest comfortably to the side and back. The body is oriented forward to ensure that your head sits parallel to your spine. Move your torso and head towards the left until you can feel a slight stretch feeling on the stretched" portion of your body. Take care not to drag your shoulders towards your ears, which is on the stretched body side instead, you should actively pull your shoulder back. Maintain your arms loose to the sides of your body. Do not bend your upper back upwards or moving the upper part of your body backwards. Move slow and slowly in a controlled method, switching parts of your body. Do this for around 1 minute.

The upper body bends in step posture.

Stand in the beginning position, extending your legs in a narrow lunge. The leg you are standing on must be bent at an angle and your front leg must be extended. Put the toes on your foot that is in front onto the flooring. Your toes face upwards. After exhaling, move your body upwards until you experience a stretching sensation on your leg's front. Keep this posture for approximately one minute while taking deep breaths in and out. You can increase the stretch feeling in the back of your bent leg by moving the body's upper part a little more in the direction of. It is possible to help the stretching with mildly springy movement in the upper part of your body. Make sure the forward leg is fully extended. After that, return to the beginning position, and repeat the exercise again on the opposite side.

Dog watching down and heel kick

In this practice, you're encouraged to bring a mat or a cushion (e.g. a yoga mat). To begin put your feet and hands onto the floor (quadruped posture). The hands should be shoulders wide and your feet should be roughly hip-width away. Then lift your buttocks to ensure that your back and arms are as straight as you can and create an even line. The buttocks are the most elevated position. Lift your feet from the floor. The legs should be slightly bent. Begin by alternating pushing your heels downwards and back to the ground. If you are unable to complete the workout for an entire time at first, you can have a break between.

Upper body stretch in lunge

In a straight position, you can lunge forward using one leg. Your weight is centered between your legs. Inhale and raise your arms upwards vertically, and stretch them to the highest point you can. While doing this, ensure that you're secure and stable until you are in the final stage of the exercise. Keep your body in the maximum stretch for only a brief time. After that, exhale and then and exhalation, you can return to your starting position and repeat the exercise. Within about a half-minute move the legs to different positions then repeat the exercise. This exercise should run for around 1 minute.

Arm sling

Standing straight, you have your legs hip-width apart with the arms are positioned alongside your body. Your head extends out the spine. Your eyes are directly in the direction of your vision. Start making small rotational movements towards the left and right. Your arms absorb the movements of your upper body. They gradually move away from you until they're nearly stretched. Slowly increase the speed of your movement. Each time, you should observe your body from behind in the most extreme rotational motion. Be sure you can freely swing your arms and your feet don't break contact with the ground as you hold your abdominals in a tight position while performing the exercise. Exercise duration: 1 minute.

5. Exercise 5" - Leg flyerFrom starting from a hip-width position and shift your body weight to one side until you are able to lift your other leg off of the floor. Begin to swing the leg in a circular motion. Then, gradually swing your arms opposite directions. The exercise helps to strengthen stabilization as well as balance at the same time. If you're confident in your technique then expand the motion range of the swing

leg. The swing leg may be a little bent through the entire swing. Make sure to swing in a forward direction and then back up as much as you can, without getting out of stability. You can then alternate your posture and swing legs. Complete the exercise in one minute.

Exercise 6 6. Heel dip

One foot should be moved further to the side as is possible in order to get an elongated foot position. You can now raise both arms up to shoulder level. Bend your upper body until your body is parallel and parallel to the flooring. Start alternating a turning movement (right/left) from your body as you shift your weight towards the leg that you're twisting your body. In parallel, bring your fingers down so that they touch the ankle of the leg to which you've shifted your weight. In parallel to this and the arm that is opposite, you should bring it up vertically until your arms create a straight horizontal line. This exercise lasts for 1 minute.

Downward-looking dog and hip twist

To perform this workout, you may make use of a cushion (e.g. a yoga mat). When you are in the beginning position put your feet and hands in the ground (quadruped position). Your hands should be about the width of your shoulders and your feet should be roughly hip width to each other. Then, raise your buttocks up vertically to ensure that your arms and back remain as straight as they can and make an even line. Your buttocks will form the top level. Then, move your buttocks in a series of steps inwards towards your feet before returning return to your starting point. In parallel to this begin a rotation of your upper body to ensure that you're able to see under your arm from the ending posture. Continue this sequence of movements for a minute.

Lateral arm swing

Your body is upright; your feet are about hip width apart and your arms hang alongside your body. Your head is extending out from your back. The gaze is directly ahead. Start to bend your torso towards the right side, in a sweep movement. Parallel to this, you can swing your left arm above your head, extending from your shoulder. The right arm is positioned in front of your body in this motion. After this, you will turn your body to your opposite side, to the left. Then, at the same time, swing your right arm upwards while lowering your left arm to your body. Repeat the movement for a full minute.

Leapfrog

To do this, you'll need an object, such as an armchair with a back that you are able to hold by your hands. The chair's seat faces away from you. Keep your hips to each other. Begin by making small vertical jumps towards the upwards. Once you're confident it is possible to perform the exercise in a safe and steady manner, you can increase the speed of your jump and then leap as high and vertically as you can. Exercise duration: 1 minute.

Interrupting jumps across the line

Your body is upright with your feet pointing at the soles of your shoes. Choose a place of reference. This could be on the floor directly in the front the feet. Then, perform quick and double-legged leaps between left and right. Think of leaping over a rope that is that is lying on the floor. Make sure you do the leaps for a minute without stopping.

Foot circles

To perform this workout for this exercise, utilize a chair, for example, holding on using only one hand. Transfer your weight on one foot and then lift one foot from the ground. Keep lifting the foot until the leg is at an 90-degree angle between the knee and the hip. Relax your hands onto your hips. Then, you will begin rotating your ankle around 15 seconds left and 15 seconds towards the right. After that, switch your legs and do this workout for a total of 15 seconds each direction.

Chapter 6: Roll, Then Sit On The Tiptoe

In a stance that is hip width in a hip-width stance, shift your body weight on one leg. Parallel to this, raise the heel of your other foot as high as you can, so that the heel of your foot reaches the floor. After that, move your heel removed from the floor back down to its starting point. You can now shift your weight on the opposite side and repeat the move. This exercise will last for 1 minute.

Exercise 1. Upper body tilt

Lift your arms in alternating upwards. Make sure you extend your hands as much as you can to either the right or left in a diagonal upward direction above your head. You should move your body in a sideways tilt and then stretch your upward body line. Your eyes should remain straight in the direction of your eyes. Your feet should be solidly planted on the ground. Do this repeatedly for around one minute.

Exercise 2 - Crossed Arm swing

Your body is straight with your hips apart and your arms hang between your legs close to your body. Your eyes are directly toward the sky. Your head extends that of the spine. Start with a few small movements of your upper part to the left and right. In parallel, you begin to pick up the motions with just one arm. While the other hand remains on the back of your body.

Increase the speed of your rotational motions And in every case take a look back at the highest potential upper body movement. The hand is extended to the position at this point and is pointing in the direction of your body. The other location, which is an reverse rotation the hand is positioned over your shoulder. You must ensure that your arm can move freely, and your feet are not losing contact with your ground. Do this for a minute.

Training 3 - Wing swing

Sit upright and keep your feet spaced hip-width separated. Bring your hands towards the floor, bending your upper body to the side. In this way, lift your arms towards the sides of your body in a way that they reach the top of your head. Next, you should move your body forward to the side and then swing" your arms back towards the sides until you get back to the beginning posture. Do this for approximately 1 minute. Make sure that you do the exercise with as much fluidity as you can.

Exercise 4: Crossing the surface of an obstruction

Imagine you're walking under a wooden slat with a height of about waist and is located on the opposite side from your back. Standing upright from the beginning position. Your feet are spaced hip-width apart and your arms hang on the sides from your body. Make a broad lunge towards the side.

Parallel to this lateral motion perform a knee bent. Move your body forward until you are approximately in line with the floor. Once you've crossed over the wooden bar, get up and return to the beginning position then repeat the exercise towards the other side. Do this for a minute.

Exercise 5 - Grow

From the beginning, your body is in the deep knee in a bend. By inhaling you, "grow" from this starting position towards the ,,sky". For this, you need to move your buttocks up vertically to make sure your legs remain straight as they can be. After that, straighten your upper back and lift your arms up.

Then, in the last position you should stand on your toes and extend your body backwards-upwards. The arms and your body make an"Y. Keep this posture for a couple of seconds prior to returning to the beginning posture and then, "growing upwards" following the time to breathe deeply. Do this for 1 minute.

Exercise 6 - Lower leg circling

If you need to, utilize a chair to hang the other hand while performing this exercise. In a stance that is hip width then shift the weight of your body on one foot and then lift your other foot off the flooring. Keep lifting the foot until the leg is at an angle of 90 degrees at the hip and knee. Set your hands to the hips. After that, you will begin rotating your lower leg, making the circular motion for 15 seconds left and 15 seconds towards the right. Switch legs, and repeat the exercise for another 15 seconds, in each direction.

Exercise 1 - Lateral lunges

Standing straight in a starting posture with your feet about hip width apart, and your hands resting between your legs. Then, bend your upper body until your body is at a level that is horizontal to the ground. Start alternating your feet towards the right or left. This exercise will last for approximately one minute.

Exercise 2 - Crossing the legs

For this workout you could employ a chair, for example, and hold onto by using just only one hand. Stand up straight and transfer the weight of your body onto one foot until you are able to take one leg off the ground.

Begin to shift your leg away from the floor left and right with the swing and behind your body. Make sure you gradually increase your swing until you achieve the maximum intensity of your motion. In about 30 seconds, repeat this exercise on the opposite leg.

Exercise 3 - Dog staring downwards, while rotating his spine

To perform this workout, you may make use of a cushion (e.g. a yoga mat). To begin you should place your feet and hands onto the floor (quadruped position). The hands are approximately shoulders wide and your feet are approximately an inch apart. Your knees may be bent. Lift your buttocks to ensure that the back and arms remain as straight as you can and make an even line. The buttocks of your body are the most elevated place to start. Now you are in the beginning position.

When you breathe out then shift your weight towards the left side of your leg, and then move your left shoulder towards the floor, the direction of parallel. The arms stay in a straight position. Your right leg helps your body stabilizes this motion and maintain your equilibrium. You should hold this position for a short time before resuming the original position by inhaling.

Perform the exercise with the other part of the body. Continue this practice until approximately 1 minute has passed.

Exercise 4 - Bend arm forward and extend into an upward lunge

Your body is in a long lunge. You are leaning your upper body toward the front, nearly in a horizontal position to the ground. After inhaling, you can start to move your arms in a forward direction and, after the exhalation, you can swing your arms backwards. As you progress, increase the force in your arms till you've reached the highest possible volume of motion.

Within 30 seconds, change the positions of your legs, placing your front foot backwards and the back leg in a forward position. Do this to complete the exercise in 1 minute.

Exercise 5 - Lower body side tilt using closed hands

Stand straight. Keep your legs more wide than the hip width and your tops of feet slightly pointing outwards while your knees are slightly bent. Place your hands over your head, so you have your fingers interlocked and your palms face upwards.

Then alternately move your body's upper part as far as is possible and right. When you're performing the move ensure that you maintain your straight torso and move as wide as you can on your side with your back facing forward. The range of motion will increase just a bit for each series of moves and complete the exercise for around one minute.

Exercise 6 - Upper body lunge bends

Stand in a tiny lunge, and then place the heel of your front foot to the ground. The feet's toes are pointed upwards. Your leg on the floor might be bent slightly. Your front leg must remain fully extended. Then, bring your chin to your chest. With the exhalation, gently lower your upper body and up, vertebra by vertebra. Reach your toes with your hand. Maintain this position for a few seconds before returning to your starting posture. Within a half-minute move your leg to a different position, then repeat the exercise on the opposite side of your body.

Exercise 1. Dog gazing down

In this type of exercise, make use of a cushion (e.g. a yoga mat). To begin you should place your feet and hands in the middle of the floor (quadruped position).

Your hands are approximately shoulders wide and your feet are approximately an inch apart. Lift your buttocks up until the back of your arms and shoulders remain as straight as they can and make an even line. The buttocks are the most prominent place to start. Lower your heels until they are on the ground. When you are in the position that you want to be your legs must be straight as they can. You should hold this position for around 1 minute.

If you're unable to complete the workout for more than more than a minute initially you can take a brief timer between sets by lying your knees down on the ground and stretching your upper body.

Exercise 2 - Arm rotation

Standing in an upright in a standing position, lift the arms towards your sides, until they are about vertical to the floor. Then begin to rotate your arms using opposite rotational motions. Your goal is to turn your hands forward and back to the maximum extent possible during every rotational movement. Do this for 1 minute.

Exercise 3 3. Alternating jumps

Sit up straight with your feet at a hip width from each other. Choose a place on the floor aligned with your feet. The point should be 20-30 inches between the feet's tops to ensure that you are in the right direction. Set one foot on your toes in this position.

Then, alternately move towards the edge using the tip of your foot and then jumping up vertically using impulsive leaps. Do this for approximately one minute, without interruptions.

Exercise 4. Double arm swing

In a standing, straight in a standing position, extend your arms up until your arms are parallel on the floor. In this position by inhaling slowly and exhalation, start to move your arms out over your back in a shoulder-length position. As you come to the finish raise your sternum a bit until you create the appearance of a hollow inside the torso.

After exhaling, bring your arms to their original posture. When you are in the right position, attempt to extend your arms towards your body to create a an incline when you reach the reverse point of the swing. While you are doing the move increase the intensity of your swings as well as the movements. In about half an hour change your foot position and repeat the exercise for the remaining 30 minutes.

Exercise 5 5. Hurdle leaps

Imagine standing an area in front of some obstacles which you'd like to jump over. Your posture is upright with your feet about the width of your hips and your arms bent. Then, you alternate lifting your knees (alternating leaps) so high as feasible using explosive pulses of jump. Utilize your arms to help support the jump and swing phases by bent at the right angles while moving them back and forth. Do this at least for one minute.

Exercise 6 - Spinning top

Standing straight with your feet separated by about a hip. Place your hands to your body and then bend your knees until you change into a squat. Start to move your arms forward of you with a variety of and circular motions. While at the same time you should return to the squat posture back to a standing posture. When your arms are over the top of your head i.e. you have reached the top the knees will be extended. Therefore, try to complete the circles as long as you can from the distance. The duration of the exercise is 1 minute.

Skater

The feet should be about an inch apart. Do a skating posture by placing your foot across the back of the other. The arm opposite of the foot placed in a backward direction performs a backward swinging motion with the arm that is bent in around right angles just in the front of your body. Return the leg placed in back into the position it was in and repeat the sequence of moves using the opposite leg and arm. Complete the whole sequence of moves with as much fluidity as you can for a minute.

Chapter 7: The Upper Body Rotates

When you are in the beginning position you're roughly hip-width apart. Your arms are hanging horizontally, parallel to each other. The arm should be bent 90 degrees, so that the forearm rests on or above the abdomen. You can put your hands in the middle of the hip on your opposite side. Inhale and raise the arm that is by bending it that is as high as you can in order to make your torso turn. Focus on the hand that is active. Your hips shouldn't move. The arm that is not active continues to rest upon your belly.

After exhaling, return the hand you are using to its starting point along the same route. Do this for around 30 seconds prior to switching sides and completing this exercise on the opposite hand.

Leg swings over an obstruction

In order to do this for this exercise, set up a stool or an obstruction about knee height to your left to provide support. The purpose of this workout is to get over an imaginary obstacle using the space between your legs. In order to do this, put your legs approximately an inch away. Then, you can swing your right leg over the imagined obstacle using an open-swinging movement left in front of you until you are able to touch the ground once more by using your right foot. After that, return the leg to its starting point using a the space-grasping motion. Once in this position continue this series of moves to the opposite side, and then repeat the whole workout for approximately 1 minute.

Standing balance

Standing upright, you shift your weight on the one leg. Lift the leg on the opposite side off the ground and then bring it to the back. In parallel, you move your upper body to the side. When you are in the position that you want, your leg and upper body create a horizontal line as close to the floor as you can. The leg that is standing may be bent slightly. The arms could be spread out to one side for the balance. The gaze must be directed towards the floor until your head aligns to your spine. Keep this posture for approximately 30 seconds before changing sideways.

Lower leg circling

In a stance with a hip width, place your weight on one foot and then lift one foot from the ground. Keep lifting this leg until the knee attains a 90-degree angle on both the hip and knee. Set your hands to the hips. Then, start to move your lower leg with the circular motion for 15 seconds left, and another 15 seconds to the right. Switch legs, and repeat the exercise for another 15 seconds, in each direction.

Exercise 1 - Bending your trunk using heel kicksPlace your feet with hip width apart in the position you started from. The arms rest on your sides, in front of your body. After exhaling, raise your chin towards your chest. Slowly bend your body, bending one vertebra at one time. Set your hands down on the ground closest to the floor as is possible. Your knees could be slightly bent when in this posture, with your heels are slightly elevated. Then, gradually raise your knees till your heels touch the level of the floor. The weight of your body is heavily on your hands throughout the movement. You are therefore stepping onto the ground, and your feet keep moving and falling off contact with the ground. It takes one minute.

Exercise 2 - Upper body stretch in lunge

In a standing, straight from a straight, upright position, make as wide an effort as you can. Your right foot is ahead, while your left foot is in the back. Your left arm is raised vertically toward the ceiling. Your right arm is still open and pointed down towards the floor. Inhale, and then move your arms upwards and backwards as much as is possible. As you stretch, make sure to maintain abdominal muscles to ensure that you're steady and safe as you get to the point where you are in the middle of this exercise. Stay in the position for a brief time. Inhale, and after that and exhalation, you can return to your starting place before shifting your foot then repeating the exercise on the opposite side of the body. The duration of the exercise is 1 minute the total.

Exercise 3. Tilt your upper body using crossed legs

Standing straight, you stand. Set your right foot behind the left side of your body in a way that the edges of your feet meet. Standing upright, you are in the beginning position for this exercise, with your legs cross-legged. After that, you should raise the right arm up vertically. Your left arm stays in your torso, and is hanging downwards vertically. Now, extend your right hand to as close as is possible up to the left side directly above your head until you experience a mild stretch on your upper right of your body. Breathe briefly and let the stretch, before exhaling and extending as much as you can up to the top left side of your head. As you move on attempt to extend slightly higher to the left while conscious exhalation to increase the length. Alternate your foot's location and repeat the movement to the opposite side of your body, for around one minute.

Exercise 4. Arm swing

Your feet should be hip-width between them. Bring both arms up towards your head. From here move your arms backwards then back to front with the greatest movement as is possible. While doing this, at the same time be sure to bend your arms and stretch your upper body downwards and towards the upwards to swing your arms. Make sure you perform space-grasping arms swings. This exercise lasts for one minute.

Exercise 5 - Arm sling

Your body is upright, with your legs hip-width apart with the arms are positioned alongside your body. Your head is extending out from your back. Your eyes are directly toward the sky. Bring your arms upwards toward the side of your body until they're placed at an even level with your flooring. Start rotating your torso in the direction of left and right. Slowly increase the speed of your movement. Each time, you should observe your body from behind in the biggest possible movement. You must ensure that your arms move freely, and that your feet are in touch with the floor. The workout should last for approximately one minute.

Training 6 - Standing up long jump

Sit upright, with your feet about hip width away. Lift both arms to the side of your head. From the starting point move your body to the side and then move your arms backwards using as wide a range of motion as is possible to begin the swinging and jumping phase. While at the same time reduce your buttocks and make a stand-up long leap forward and upwards using as much force as feasible. Perform 10 jumps.

Exercise 1: Upper body is bent by rotating

Your feet should be hip-width to each other. The arms rest on your sides, in front of your body. Keep your chin in your chest. From this point and exhale, gently bend your upper body downwards, vertebra by vertebra. Make sure to extend your fingers in the direction of the ground.

Then, while in this position move your body towards the right to move the left hand towards the right side of your foot. After that, turn your upper body towards the left in order to be able to transfer your right hand to the left side of your foot. Straighten your upper body and repeat this exercise with a brief stop. Perform this exercise again at a slow and controlled move until one minute is up.

Exercise 2 - Alternate tilts in the body's upper part

Stand straight with your feet firmly pressed together. Your arms are relaxed between your legs close to your body. Then, you face forward to ensure that your spine and head create one straight line. Then, stretch your upper body towards the other side until you can feel a slight stretch sensation in the, "stretched" part of the body. You must ensure that you do not push your shoulders towards your ears while you stretch the side of your body instead, you should push" your shoulder downwards. Maintain your arms loose to the sides of your body. Be careful not to bend your upper body towards the front or pushing the upper part of your body backwards.

You should perform this move slow and slowly in a controlled method, switching side of the body. Perform this exercise for approximately 1 minute.

Exercise 3 - Leg flyer

In this workout, you could make use of a chair and (writing) table to provide assistance. With a hip-width stance transfer your weight on one foot until you're able to raise the other leg off the ground. Start swinging your free leg forward and back. Parallel to this, you can swing your upper body in a circular motion. Slowly swing your arms in opposite directions. The exercise helps to strengthen stabilization and balance at the exact time. When you are secure, expand the motion range of the swing leg. Your leg on the ground is supposed to be bent slightly during the swing. You should try to swing upwards and forwards return up as high as you can, without falling off stability. You can then alternate the stance as well as swinging leg. Complete the exercise in 1 minute.

Exercise 4 - Balancing

In order to complete the exercise you'll need the object you want to use like a ball you are able to balance with your hands. Standing up with your legs hip-width apart. Place the object you want to hold in your hands and place it up to your chest at a at a level. Another, passive" arm is positioned across your body. Move your "active" arm in the direction of the object up and forward until the arm extends. Move your hands along an imaginary line that is U-shaped past your body to the hip level and then rotate your upper body towards the object, and then move your hands back up until the arm is extended yet again. The upper part of your body is turned towards the front and bent slightly at this point. After a few seconds and then move the arm back to the original position. Switch sides, and repeat the same movement using your opposite hand. Exercise duration: 1 minute.

Exercise 5 Exercise 5 Diagonal crunch

Standing upright, shift your weight on the one leg. You can place the opposite leg behind you and rest your feet on the floor. In parallel, lift the opposite arm up to the height of your head. Begin by bringing the knee of your leg that is behind you, as well as the elbow of your opposite arm in the front of your torso, until they are in a position to touch. After that, return to the beginning posture before repeating the move. The exercise should last for around 30 seconds for each part of the body.

Exercise 6 - Overstep

Standing straight, shift the weight of your body onto the one leg. The other leg is moved to the opposite side of your body by taking a step in a slack direction backwards by lifting your leg as high as you can. Once you have placed your foot in the ground, return your leg back to its starting posture using the same method.

Chapter 8: Planning Is Half The Battle

In the initial chapters you've learned that paying taking care of the fascia is crucial when you are looking to do things to improve your health and overall health. The fascia's changes are slow, but it is true that consistent and lasting - longer-lasting fascia care can lead to an improvement of the structure of fascia. It does not matter when you first begin to train. All you need is begin.

However, starting out isn't too difficult It's persistence which is the issue. This isn't for everyone however, for many. You might also be part of the majority group with an extremely dominant, "inner animal" which keeps us from making best resolutions. You can outwit the "inner the pig" by employing a few strategies this time.

Create realistic targets!

The Roman poet and philosopher Seneca is often quoted in this context, and states, mutatis mutandis If a sailer doesn't decide which beach to go to, no wind will be appropriate." This means that you must to determine where you wish to go, so that you are able to decide the best way in order to reach your goal. What is your goal? The destination you choose could be like:

I want to lessen my neck and back discomfort over the next three months."

One of the best things to do is to grab an old piece of paper or use a notebook app to note down the goals you want to achieve. If you've undergone hip surgery, you might focus more on the goal of reducing hip discomfort. Make sure you write down the objective, and don't get distracted from the goal. For instance, you can place the sheet of paper at your desk or hang it in your kitchen, or keep your electronic notes displayed daily on your mobile at the beginning of your day.

Think about the benefits!

Relax your eyes and think that you've accomplished the goal you set for yourself. What changes have been made for you? For instance:

less discomfort in the neck and back region.

less stress

greater ability to concentrate

improved general well-being

All in all, you'll improve your overall quality of life which is worth giving up just a bit of time to achieve that goal, isn't it? Put the results on your page of paper and on your smartphone.

Operate consistent risk management!

Have you tried before to shed weight by following eating a strict diet, or by doing more exercise? Do you recognize the reasons that cause initiatives to boost your health not succeed: limited time appointment reminders or too hard, the fear of embarrassing yourself, an appetite for food and temptations from the fridge as well as, in. It is worth taking time time to think about the factors that may hinder you from getting your regular exercise into. Add to your notes goal making and consider the advantages of your new exercise routine as well as the possible risks. Consider how you could deal with the risk.

We've already aided our clients with regard to the most common risk:

The workout programs run just 7 minutes.

The exercises are not requiring any other equipment

The exercise programs are very simple

The exercise program is dependent,

The workout programmes do not require sporting attire,

The exercise routines can be completed at home or at work.

Our focus is on the low threshold for a greater chance of you completing an hour-long daily routine for you and your overall health. Why do you need to exercise daily? We believe it is more convenient to establish the daily routine to exercise routine regularly. This could be early in the morning, following waking up, at the office, before heading to the cafeteria at night, or as you watch the television news.

You can measure your success!

Did you complete your health-related personal project? When you've attained or exceeded your target in the designated time! Take the following illustration above to illustrate the goal. "I'd prefer to reduce significantly my shoulder and back pain in three months."

You want to determine the extent to which the pain in your neck and back decreases. Because this is an subjective feeling It is a smart option to utilize the pain questionnaire as a measurement tool. If you don't have a pain questionnaire in your possession or you want to download one, then you can find the sample of a pain questionnaire by visiting the download page to use for your assessment of the efficacy in self-treatment.

Pain area	Pain intensity									
	no	weak			moderate			strong		very strong
Head	0	1	✕	3	4	5	6	7	8	9	10
Neck/Shoulder	0	1	2	3	4	5	6	7	✕	9	10
Cross/Back	0	1	2	3	4	✕	6	7	8	9	10
Elbow, right	✕	1	2	3	4	5	6	7	8	9	10
Elbow, left	✕	1	2	3	4	5	6	7	8	9	10
Wrist, right	✕	1	2	3	4	5	6	7	8	9	10
Wrist, left	✕	1	2	3	4	5	6	7	8	9	10

You can base your decision upon a specific amount of time such as the past four weeks. In the event that you experience extreme pain in your neck or shoulder region, you can enter an "8" in this field. If you experience moderately intense pain in your back region, give the number,4" or ,,5" for the back location.

According to the goals formulation, you should attain "significant" alleviation of pain by treatment of the fasciae. What exactly does "significant" refers to? The answer is you can decide for yourself. Example: in the shoulder and neck area You want to increase your range of motion by reducing the number of,,8" to ,,5", which is to go back down from "severe" to ,,moderate" pain. In the back, pain part isn't as intense. In this case, you should aim to reduce the pain from, 5" (,,moderate" pain) to, 3" (,,low" pain). It is important to make your form more specific, in light of these aspects:

I'd like to lower my shoulder/neck pain from 8" to ,,5" and my back pain, which is ranging from 5" to ,,3" in the coming three months."

Therefore, you must make the first measurement prior to starting the fascia treatment (then you can determine from which point the ship will begin) After three months, you will take another measurement (then you will know when your ship has landed). The next step is of knowing how you'll arrive at your final destination.

If you are new treating fascia issues, you must begin with the "Basic program" and then gradually integrate the ,,Strong Back Program" and the "Fit Back Program". You might decide to reserve 7 minutes for treatment of the fascia each morning at the conclusion of your work day or while watching the news on TV at night. The treatment program could be like this such as:

1st measurement: pain questionnaire (PQJ14-G)

1. First week BASIC PROGRAM

2nd Week: BASIC PROGRAM

3-week week Strong BACK

4th week STRONGER BACK

5th week 5th week: FIT BACK

6th week of FIT BACK

*7th week BASIC PROGRAM STONG BACK (in alternate)

8. BASIC PROGRAM and STRONG BACK (in the order of)

9. BASIC PROGRAM, BACK FIT (in alternate)

*10th week BASIC PROGRAM. FIT BACK (in alternate)

11. BASIC PROGRAM. STRONG BACK and BACK FIT (in the order of)

The 12th week is BASIC PROGRAM, STONG BACK AND Fit BACK (in the order of)

2nd measurement: pain questionnaire (PQJ14-G)

The measurement results will be evaluated as well as your own experience. a new setting of goals with the adapted treatment plan.

Develop an action plan and start moving!

The treatment plan should be transferred to your calendar. You can set the date of the initial measurement as well as your second one. Set aside 7 minutes per day on your calendar to you, to do the treatment of your fascia. It is best to arrange your workout timings in exactly the same time of day, when you can.

If you're ever unable to attend any self-care or" several sessions because you aren't able to make it happen Don't let it discourage you. The same thing happens over and over time and time again. Start your new program or resume from where you started. The one thing you must be avoiding is throwing in the towel" and putting your efforts for your own health ,,ad acta".

Get support from other people. Perhaps you have a friend who is also looking to make a difference for his or her well-being. Participate in the program together or discuss if you've taken or stopped taking self-care.

Chapter 9: A Case For Load Training

The practice of lagging, also referred to as resistance training is an training that involves lifting weights, or any other form of resistance, in order to improve strength and strength and muscle mass. Training with weights has lots benefits not only for general health but also to achieve specific goals like growing muscle mass or improving the performance of athletes.

One of the primary advantages of training with loads is its capacity to boost the strength of muscles and increase their size. Since muscles have to endure greater levels of force as they grow, they become more powerful and bigger with time. This could lead to better endurance, improved bone density, as well as a decreased risk of injuries.

Training for weights can improve heart health as it may improve lung and heart function as well as improve the body's capacity to make use of oxygen.

Furthermore, it's proven to increase insulin sensitivity as well as blood sugar control. This could help reduce the likelihood of getting type 2 diabetes.

Training for load can improve the mental wellbeing. It's been proven to help reduce the symptoms of depression and anxiety as well as improve cognitive performance and boost overall sense of happiness.

In the end, the advantages of weight training makes it a crucial component in any fitness program. It's an efficient method to boost the strength of athletes, their athletic ability, as well as general health and wellbeing.

Chapter 10: The Anatomy Of Pain

It is a painful sensation which can result from different factors like injuries, illnesses, or even inflammation. The understanding of the anatomy that causes pain will help identify the root of the discomfort and develop efficient treatment methods.

The body's nervous system is an important role in the feeling of discomfort. In the event of any kind of tissue injury, specific nerve fibers, known as nociceptors, are activated. They transmit information regarding the damage or injury through the spinal cord as well as the brain, which can be perceived as a feeling of pain.

There are two kinds of pain: acute or chronic. The term "cute" refers to a brief feeling that happens due to an occasion, for instance, an injury or broken bone. Chronic pain however it is a longer-lasting sensation which lasts longer than 3 months. Chronic pain may be caused through a myriad of causes, like chronic damaged nerves, or diseases.

The severity of pain may differ widely based upon the severity of the injury, or another factors that cause the inflammation. The intensity of pain can be affected by different factors, such as the individual's mood as well as their stress levels as well as their past experiences dealing with pain.

Through understanding the anatomy of discomfort and the various elements which can cause it, health professionals are able develop efficient treatment plans to alleviate pain and increase your quality of life patients suffering from pain.

Fascia is a form of connective tissue which surrounds and supports muscles, bones, as well as organs of the body. It's made of collagen fibers. It can be all over the body, beginning at the top of your head down to the top of toes.

Fascia has a significant role within the body's musculoskeletal system and helps provide the body with stability and support. the body. When fascia gets too tight or restricted this can cause stiffness and pain in the joints.

The tightness of the fascia could cause imbalances and misalignment in the joints causing discomfort and stiffness. Additionally, it can affect the normal functioning of muscles, resulting in decreased mobility and flexibility. In some instances it is possible that tight fascia be a contributing factor to in the development of chronic pain disorders.

In contrast an elongated and healthy fascia can be flexible and elastic, which allows the body to move in a fluid and easily. When you keep your fascia in good condition, you will increase your health and flexibility in the musculoskeletal system as well as reduce stiffness and pain as well as improve general flexibility and mobility.

The role of fascia during pain can be multi-faceted. The tightness or restriction of fascia could cause pain and discomfort, but good fascia health can alleviate pain and enhance general musculoskeletal wellness.

Chapter 11: What To Concentrate On Rather Than Pain Relief

Instead of just focusing on relieving pain It can be beneficial to focus also on the root of the problem in order to promote overall wellness and health. There are some things to think about:

The root of the pain. Rather than dealing with the pain's symptoms It is far more efficient to focus on what is causing the suffering. It could involve collaborating with a health professional in order to identify and treat related health problems or injuries that contribute to the discomfort.

Be mindful of the overall wellbeing and health A healthy and balanced lifestyle helps to delay the beginning of pain as well as improve the general quality of life. This could mean having a balanced diet as well as regular exercise as well as managing anxiety.

Find coping strategies that are healthy and effective The chronic pain condition can be an extremely difficult condition to deal with. It is essential to discover the most effective ways to deal with the pain by practicing mindfulness, engaging in exercising, or getting the support of family and friends.

Consider physical therapy, or alternative forms of rehabilitation The use of physical therapy as well as other rehabilitation methods can assist in enhancing the strength, flexibility and mobility. This will in turn assist in reducing pain.

Focusing on these issues instead of just pain relief You can adopt an approach that is more holistic in managing your pain, and improve overall health and wellbeing.

Here are some concrete ways you can concentrate on repairing your fascia, instead of just looking for the relief you need:

Make use of self-myofascial releases: Self-myofascial releases like foam rolling, are a great way in releasing tight fascia and increase mobility.

Do regular stretching: Regularly stretching helps maintain a healthy fascia that is elastic, decreasing the chance of injuries and increasing the overall flexibility.

Keep hydrated: Proper hydration is crucial to maintain a good health of your fascia. Drink ample amounts of water and other fluids to ensure that your fascia well-hydrated and working correctly.

Maintain a good posture. Good position can reduce tension on the muscles as well as fascia, which can prevent tension and dysfunction.

You may want to consider working with a therapy professional The physical therapist will aid you in identifying any misalignments or imbalances throughout your body. He can develop an individual treatment plan to enhance your health of the fascia and ease the pain.

Focusing on these simple ways, you'll be able to adopt a an active approach to improving the condition of your fascia as well as reducing discomfort, instead of relieving yourself on methods to relieve pain.

Chapter 12: How To Train Your Collagen

Fascia is a form of connective tissue which surrounds and supports muscles, bones, as well as organs of the body. It's made of collagen fibers. It is located throughout the body beginning at the top of your head all the way to the tip of toes.

The connection between collagen and fascia is the fact that collagen is the main element of the fascia. The collagen fibers provide assistance and support to fascia, assisting keep its strength and structural integrity. They also help to function correctly.

There are several methods to help assist in promoting the health and production of collagen throughout your body. These will in turn help to improve the function and health of your fascia.

Consume a diet rich in collagen: A few foods high in collagen or help in collagen production are seafood, bone broth and leaves of greens, as well as fruit that are that are high in Vitamin C.

Find enough protein Collagen can be described as a protein therefore it is important to make sure you're taking in enough protein through your diet in order to aid collagen production. Protein sources that are good include chicken, meat, fish as well as beans and nuts.

Utilize collagen supplements: Collagen supplements, like collagen peptides, or collagen powder can be added to your food in order to help boost the production of collagen.

Guard your skin against UV harm: UV radiation can damage the collagen that is present in your skin, which can cause wrinkles, as well as other signs of the aging process. By wearing sunscreen and a protective garment, you will help shield the skin against UV harm and help maintain your collagen health.

Regular exercise has been proven to boost collagen synthesis as well as improve the durability and strength of the connective tissues.

If you follow these guidelines follow these suggestions, you can help aid in the growth and maintenance of collagen throughout your body. You can also maintain the integrity and strength of your fascia as well as other connective tissues.

Below is a listing of food items that are high in collagen, or support collagen production

Bone broth Bone broth is an excellent supply of collagen, along with other minerals that aid in the production of collagen, like amino acids as well as minerals.

Seafood: Seafoods, specifically shellfish is an excellent source of collagen-supporting nutrients, such as proline and glycine.

Green leafy vegetables like kale, spinach as well as broccoli are abundant in minerals and vitamins which help collagen synthesizing.

Fruits rich in vitamin C: Vitamin C is crucial for collagen production, and citrus fruits like strawberry, oranges and kiwifruits are rich in the nutrient.

Yellow and red peppers They are rich in vitamin C, as well as other minerals which aid collagen production.

Garlic: Garlic contains compounds which may aid collagen synthesis as well as defend collagen against damage.

Tomatoes: Tomatoes can be an excellent source of lycopene. It is an antioxidant, which may aid to shield collagen from harm.

When you incorporate these rich collagen-rich foods to your daily diet, you will be able to support the growth and well-being of collagen within your body. It is important to keep in mind that collagen supplements could provide support for collagen production, but their effectiveness has not been proven.

CHAPTER5

Movement: The Original Mobility

The movement is the primary type of movement and is vital to human well-being and overall health. From the moment we're born, we play an important role in our development and helps us develop, learn and learn about our environment.

The movement can come in many kinds, like dancing, walking, running or swimming. It could be conscious and conscious activity. And it is a vital part of living a healthy and balanced lifestyle.

The benefits of exercise are many and numerous. Exercise can boost cardiovascular health, enhance endurance and flexibility of the muscles, as well as maintain an ideal weight. Also, it has positively impact on your mental health by reducing anxiety and stress, as well as increasing cognitive and mood.

Apart from these benefits moving is essential to maintain good health of the fascia and connective tissues. Through regular exercise and participation in various exercises, you will assist in keeping your fascia flexible and healthy which will reduce the possibility of stiffness, pain, and so on.

In the end it is true that movement is the primary type of mobility that is crucial for wellbeing and health. When you incorporate a range of exercises into your daily routine it is possible to benefit from the many benefits of exercise and also maintain good health for your connective tissues.

There are various types of exercises that will assist in keeping your fascia flexible and healthy. Here are a few of them:

Walking It is an easy and efficient method to boost your general mobility as well as ensure that your fascia stays healthy. Begin by taking about 30 minutes every day. Gradually increase your distance as you get more at ease.

Stretching out regularly: It helps keep your fascia supple and decrease the chance of stiffness and discomfort. Consider incorporating several stretch routines into your routine by focusing on the different muscles.

Yoga The practice of yoga that consists of stretching and postures which can increase flexibility and improve mobility. Yoga poses are often focused on lengthening and stretching the fascia, which makes it a great alternative to improve the health of fascia.

Swimming It is a non-impact activity that is able to increase flexibility and mobility overall. The buoyancy in the water assists in supporting the body, which allows people to move around freely and in a comfortable way.

Resistance training: Resistance exercises including weight lifting or bodyweight exercise, may aid in improving endurance and strength and, in turn, aid in maintaining strong fascia.

If you're just beginning to learn about these exercises, you can try to incorporate these into your daily routine. Begin by doing shorter workouts then gradually increase duration and intensity once you're more at ease. You must pay attention to your body's signals and stop whenever there is any discomfort or discomfort.

When you incorporate a variety of activities in your routine it will help maintain your fascia's health and supple, decreasing your risk of suffering from pain and stiffness.

Chapter 13: Science-Backed Mobility Training

The practice of mobility training is one type of workout that concentrates on increasing range of motion for joints as well as flexibility and mobility. It is a great method to lessen discomfort, enhance fitness levels, and improve the overall quality and function of living.

There are a variety of methods of training for mobility, and the most effective method is dependent on the specific needs and goals of yours. Below are some scientifically-based methods for implementing the training for mobility:

Utilize self-myofascial release techniques Self-myofascial releases like foam rolling, may help to ease tightness and restrict within the fascia, and increase general mobility.

Regularly stretch: It is a vital part of the training for mobility as it can improve mobility and flexibility. Integrate a variety of stretching exercises in your routine and concentrate on the different joint and muscle groups.

Make use of dynamic stretching, which involves the active movement, can be more efficient in strengthening your mobility than static stretches. Think about incorporating dynamic stretching in your routine for example, the shoulder circle or leg swings.

Utilize progressive overload: It is a method which involves gradually increasing the difficulty or intensity of the training for mobility over time. It can be helpful to continually enhance your mobility and stop plateaus.

Get a professional coach or physical therapist or physical therapist may assist you in creating an individual mobility program which is tailored to your requirements and objectives. They are also able to provide direction and advice for you to make improvements and prevent injuries.

With these proven strategies to implement mobility training to enhance your overall mobility and performance.

Here are some useful strategies for implementing scientifically-supported movement training

Begin slowly. When beginning the new program of mobility it is essential to begin with a slow pace and then gradually increase intensities. This can help you keep from injury while giving the body time to adjust to the changes in demands.

Make use of a variety of strategies Utilizing a range of training methods for mobility including the stretching of foam rolls and dynamic exercises, will assist to provide an all-encompassing strategy for increasing mobility.

Be aware of your posture Correct posture is vital while performing any mobility exercises. Be sure to adhere to the correct method and stop whenever there is any discomfort or discomfort.

Be sure to breathe properly. Correct breathing practices can assist to increase mobility and decrease tension on the body. If you are doing exercises to improve mobility make sure you are breathing slowly and deeply.

Integrate mobility-related training in your everyday routine For the maximum benefit from your the practice of mobility, you need to integrate it as a part of your daily routine. Set the time throughout the day to work on your mobility, regardless of whether that's in the early hours of the morning, or prior to going to you go to bed.

If you follow these strategies, you'll be able to implement a scientifically-based training in mobility to improve your overall performance and mobility. Always listen to your body's signals and stop when there is any discomfort or discomfort. Also, be aware to seek advice from an expert in your medical field if there are any issues.

CHAPTER7

Corrective Routines

Corrective exercises are actions that are created to target specific weaknesses or body dysfunction. They're often utilized to increase mobility, decrease discomfort, and enhance the overall performance.

In order to carry out the corrective procedures successfully, it is essential to initially identify the particular issues or imbalances you're trying to correct. It may require working with a medical professional like physical therapist, to determine the root cause of any problems.

When you've pinpointed the particular imbalance or problem that you wish to correct, you may decide on certain exercises or moves which are specifically designed to fix those problems. The exercises could involve strengthening, stretching, or mobility exercises, and could be accomplished using bodyweight as well as resistance bands or any other piece of devices.

Regular exercises that correct the imbalance can be beneficial for the health of your fascia, since they are able to enhance mobility and flexibility, lessen stiffness and pain, as well as help to prevent injuries. When you address specific imbalances or issues, you'll assist in keeping your fascia strong and healthy.

For the greatest benefit from your corrective regimens It is essential to remain regular and have them become routinely component in your routine. Also, it's important to pay attention to your body's signals and immediately stop when you notice discomfort or pain or to speak with an expert in your healthcare in case you are concerned.

There are numerous types of routines for correcting imbalances which can be utilized to correct particular imbalances or issues throughout the body. These are just a few of them:

Stretching: It is an integral part of routines that correct posture, because it aids in improving range of motion and flexibility. For a successful stretch, you must hold the stretch for a minimum of 30 seconds while focusing on breathing slowly and deeply.

Exercises for strengthening: Strengthening including squats, or lunges, are a great way to build endurance and strength that can then aid in maintaining healthy fascia and connective tissues. In order to perform these exercises efficiently ensure you are using the correct technique. begin with a low amount of weight or resistance. Then, you can increase them the strength you gain.

Mobility drills: Mobility exercises that include shoulders circles or leg swings could be utilized to enhance the range of motion and flexibility. For a successful performance of these exercises concentrate on fluid precise movements. You should stop whenever you feel any discomfort or pain.

Foam rolling It is a kind of self-myofascial release method which can be utilized to relieve tightness and restrictions within the fascia. To effectively foam roll you need to apply moderate pressure the muscle or tissue you wish to target as you roll around at a steady pace.

Chapter 14: Preventing The Big Three

"Big Three "Big Three" are common muscular and skeletal injuries which can lead to stiffness, pain and diminished mobility. The three types of injuries are:

Lower back pain or low back pain is an atypical condition that is result of a myriad of reasons, like the imbalance of muscles, poor posture and excessive use.

Knee pain The pain in the knee is caused by various issues, such as tendonitis, arthritis and injuries to ligaments.

Shoulder pain Shoulder pain could be result of a range of problems, such as bursitis, rotator cuff injury as well as tendinitis.

To avoid getting from developing the Big Three, it's important to keep a focus on maintaining general musculoskeletal wellness. Below are some methods that may assist:

Be sure to maintain a healthy weight. The extra weight you carry can cause additional strain on your muscular system, increasing the chance of getting injured. A healthy weight will aid in reducing the risk.

Regularly exercising helps to increase the strength of your muscles, flexibility and mobility, thus reducing the chance of sustaining injuries.

Maintain a good posture. Good posture will help reduce the chance of injuries to your musculoskeletal system by helping in distributing your weight evenly and reduce strain on certain joints or muscles.

Keep hydrated. Dehydration could cause discomfort and stiffness which can increase the chance of an injury. Be sure to drink plenty of fluids throughout the day to remain well-hydrated.

Make sure you wear appropriate footwear that is comfortable and is supportive of your feet will aid in reducing the chance of injury to your musculoskeletal structure.

With these methods using these tips, you can keep away from The Big Three and maintain good overall health of your musculoskeletal system.

There are numerous types of workout routines that assist in the prevention of from developing the Big Three and maintain good overall health of the musculoskeletal system. Here are some of them:

Strength training: Strength-training exercises, like lunges and squats, may assist in enhancing endurance and strength and reduce the chance of injuries. For effective performance of these exercises ensure you are using the right technique. begin with a low amount of weight or resistance. Then, you can increase them when you get stronger.

Yoga It is a form of exercise that includes a set of stretching and poses which can enhance flexibility and mobility. A lot of yoga postures focus on strengthening and stretching joints and muscles. This makes yoga a great option to avoid from the Big Three.

Pilates: Pilates is a kind of exercise which focuses on strengthening core muscles, and improving general stability and stability. Pilates can be a beneficial method to avoid getting the Big Three and improve musculoskeletal well-being.

Exercise that is cardiovascular like running or cycling, may help in improving cardiovascular health as well as lower the chance of developing muscular injuries.

For the greatest benefit from these workout routines It is essential to remain regular and have them become routinely component in your routine. It's equally important to pay attention to your body, and then immediately stop when you notice any discomfort or pain as well as to talk an expert in your healthcare if there's any concern.

Chapter 15: Injury Recovery: Strategy And Tactics

The procedure of returning to normal functioning and normal activity following the occurrence of an injury. This can be a complicated process, however, with proper strategies and techniques you can complete a full recovery.

A key element of recovering from injuries is creating plans for your rehabilitation. It should be personalized to the specific injuries and needs, and could include a mix of physical therapy, exercises as well as other treatments.

A key aspect in healing from injuries is addressing the inflammation and pain. It can involve the use of heat or ice, medication over the counter or prescribed and alternative therapies including massage, acupuncture, or acupressure.

It's equally important to keep an eye on proper nutrition when you are in healing. A balanced diet with plenty of nutrients will aid in healing and rehabilitation.

In the end, it's essential to take your time and be consistent when it comes to your recovery plan. There is a temptation to put yourself in a hurry or try to resume normal activities at a rapid pace, but it could actually hinder your recovery. If you follow a regular and well-planned recovery plan and implementing an entire recovery, and then return to your normal routine.

Below are some practical methods you could employ for quick recovery from injury:

Make sure you follow a regular rehabilitation program You must follow the same rehabilitation schedule specific to the specific injuries you have and objectives. This could involve exercise as well as physical therapy or various other treatments.

Control inflammation and pain: In order to manage inflammation and pain you can try ice and warmth, using over-the counter or prescription medicines, or alternatives to treatments like massage or acupuncture.

A well-balanced and balanced diet is recommended: An energizing and balanced diet full of nutrients could assist in recovery and healing. Concentrate on eating lots of fresh fruits, vegetables and protein that is lean Avoid refined and sweet foods.

Drink plenty of water: Hydration is essential for the recovery of injuries because it assists in helping eliminate toxins and aid in the healing process. Drink plenty of fluids throughout your entire day.

Sleep enough: Proper sleep is crucial for the recovery of injuries. It is important to ensure you have a restful night's sleep each night, and stay clear of things that could aggravate the injuries.

If you follow these techniques, you can help rapid recovery from injuries and get back to your normal activities as quickly as you can.

Make sure to pay attention to your body's signals and cease exercise whenever you notice any pain or discomfort. Make aware to seek advice from an expert in your healthcare in case you are concerned.

Chapter 16: Exercise Programming And Periodization

Periodization and programming for exercise is the procedure of creating and arranging an exercise routine that will help you achieve specific targets. This involves breaking your workout program into smaller, easier to manage pieces, known as "periods," and varying the volume, intensity and intensity of your exercise throughout time.

There are numerous ways to approach exercise programming and periodicization. The most effective approach is dependent on your particular desires and goals. A few common methods include:

Linear periodization Linear periodization is the gradual increase in intensity of your training over time beginning with lower intense workouts before progressing to more intense workouts.

Non-linear Periodization: Non-linear periodicity means that you can alter the volume, intensity and intensity of your exercises in a way that is more random and not using a specific pattern.

Undulating Periodization: Undulating means that you are constantly varying the intensity and concentration of your training instead of having a specific pattern of progression.

With the help of exercise programs and a timer, you will be able to efficiently plan and arrange your training sessions to meet your desired objectives. This helps to avoid the occurrence of plateaus, and also help improve your progress overall.

Why It's Smart to Be Disciplined

Becoming disciplined involves being consistent in executing your promises and making choices to help you achieve your long-term objectives. Being disciplined is a smart choice as it will help you achieve your goals and achieve your goals more swiftly and effectively.

Here are a few of the reasons for why it's a good idea to stay controlled:

The discipline of discipline helps you stay in the present: If you're well-organized, you are able to focus on your objectives and avoid distractions that may distract you from your goal. This helps you keep moving towards your goal and be successful faster.

The discipline of discipline helps you manage your time efficiently: When you are well-organized, you are able to control your time efficiently and avoid the waste of time doing things that don't help your objectives. This will allow you to accomplish more with less time and make more efficient use of the resources you have.

It helps to develop positive habits. Through staying disciplined, you'll be able to develop positive habits that will help your objectives and set the stage for your the success you desire. These can be things such like exercising frequently as well as eating healthy meals as well as managing your money successfully.

It helps to conquer obstacles: Being disciplined will assist you to remain engaged and focused facing obstacles or backslides. This will help you be resilient and overcome challenges which could otherwise hinder your efforts.

If you are disciplined by being disciplined, you will ensure that you are on the right track and accomplish your goals rapidly and effectively.

Chapter 17: Getting The Motions Right

Making sure that the movements are correct is essential to many tasks, such as exercises, sports, as well as everyday chores. When motions are done correct, they will be more effective, efficient and safe. If the movements are done incorrectly, they could be more inefficient, less safe, and even more dangerous.

Here are some tips to ensure you are doing the right motions:

Attention to your posture Attention to the form is vital for any movement. Always follow the proper procedure and stay clear of any moves that make you feel uncomfortable or uncomfortable.

Prioritize quality over the quantity of motions: when performing exercises It is important to concentrate on the quality of your work, not the quantity. Instead of rushing through the motions be sure to make sure to take time and take the time to do each by paying attention and care to the smallest of details.

Make sure you are using proper equipment is a way to make sure that you're doing the movements correctly and in a safe manner. It could include wearing appropriate shoes as well as gloves and other gear to protect yourself.

Get advice from a professional If you're not sure about how to execute an action correctly, get assistance from a qualified. The person you seek guidance from could be a coach or instructor, or a healthcare specialist, based on your task at hand.

If you follow these guidelines You can increase your performance and lower the likelihood of injuries. This will help you become more effective, efficient and safe when you perform your tasks.

Mobility, Core, and Dynamic Warm-up

An ad hoc, core and dynamic warm-up one type of exercise routine which is intended to get your body ready to perform physical activities. The typical approach is a mix of the core exercise, and active stretching that are designed to increase flexibility, stability and strength.

Here are some examples of core, mobility and dynamic warm-ups:

Mobility exercises: These exercises aim to increase flexibility as well as mobility in joints. Examples are lunges and hip swings, or shoulder circles.

Core exercises: Core workouts are intended to build the muscles that make up the trunk as well as improve the stability of your body. Examples of this include side planks, as well as bird dogs.

Dynamic stretch: Dynamic stretches can be stretches performed through movement as opposed to static stretches that are performed in a fixed place. Examples are leg swings, high knees and butt kicks.

Conducting a flexibility, core as well as dynamic warm-up could assist in getting your body ready to perform physical activities, lessen your risk of injuries, and increase your overall performance. It is generally suggested to do warming up routine prior to engaging in any physical workout as well as sports and daily chores.

In order to perform a core, mobility energetic, or core warm-up, you must follow these steps:

Begin by doing mobility exercises Begin with a set of movements that improve the flexibility as well as range of motion the joints. For example, lunges, hip swings, shoulders circles, and leg swings. Do each exercise for about 10 repetitions for each side.

Incorporate core exercise Then, add the core exercise routine to build the strength of the trunk as well as improve the stability. Some examples include side planks and planks as well as bird dogs. Each exercise should be performed for 10 repetitions per side.

Follow with a series of dynamic stretches. Then, finish the warm-up exercise with a sequence of stretches that are dynamic to increase flexibility as well as prepare muscles for moving. Some examples include leg swings, high knees and butt kicks. Each stretch should be performed for 10 repetitions per side.

It's recommended that you perform the warm-up routine between 5 and 10 minutes prior to any exercise. This will help prepare your body to handle the demands of your activity as well as reduce the possibility of injury and increase your overall performance. Make sure to pay attention to your body's signals and to stop when there is any discomfort or discomfort.

Shoulder Stability

Stability of the shoulder is the ability that the shoulder joint has in maintaining the correct balance and strength when performing activities. A stable shoulder is essential when performing activities that require the upper part of your body, for example, lifting, pushing and pulling. It can reduce the chance of injury, and also improve performance.

There are a variety of aspects that could influence shoulder stability, like muscle strength, flexibility and control. Here are a few suggestions which can aid in improving shoulder stability

The shoulder muscles should be strengthened By strengthening the muscles of the shoulders specifically the rotator cuff muscles, may help increase the stability of your shoulder. It can be accomplished through exercises like shoulder presses or lateral lifts as well as exercise for the rotator-cuff.

Increase flexibility by increasing flexibility of the shoulder muscles as well as the surrounding joints helps enhance the stability of your shoulder. This is possible with stretching exercises, such as shoulders stretches as well as chest stretches.

A good and healthy posture position can strengthen the shoulder by putting the spine and shoulders into the correct posture. Be sure to stand up and sit straight and stay clear of hunching over.

Utilizing the correct technique while performing exercises for the upper body can assist in improving the stability of your shoulders. Always use your arms and shoulders to lift objects in an upright and stable position to avoid straining your shoulders or reaching out too high.

With these techniques by following these strategies, you will improve your shoulder strength and decrease risk of injuries when performing activities that require movements of the upper body.

There are many theories regarding the best way to perform exercises for shoulder stability to increase shoulder stability, and lessen the chance of sustaining injuries. Below are some examples:

Theory of Progressive Overload Based on the progressive overload concept, the ideal method to increase shoulder stability is gradually increasing intensities of workouts throughout time. This could be accomplished by increasing the weight resistance or the number of repetitions you do your exercises or even by reducing the interval between sets.

Specificity theory: The theory states that the most efficient method to increase the stability of your shoulder is to focus on exercises specifically targeting the muscles of the shoulder and its adjacent joints. It could include exercises that target the shoulder like a shoulder press or lateral lifts as well as the rotator cuff exercises.

Theory of individual differences Individual differences theory indicates that the ideal method to strengthen shoulder strength could differ based on the particular person's individual characteristics including fitness level, age, and medical background. This theory highlights the importance of adjusting exercise plans to each person's individual requirements and objectives.

Neural adaptation theory The theory of neural adaptation suggests that the ideal method to increase shoulder stability could be to increase the coordination and control of neural systems of shoulder muscles. This could be accomplished by doing exercises that test stabilization and balance, for instance exercises with a single arm or on surfaces that are unstable.

If you think about these ideas in addition to focusing on the exercises and methods suitable for your particular goals and requirements it is possible to improve shoulder strength and decrease the likelihood of injuries.

For exercises to strengthen your shoulder to improve shoulder stability adhere to these guidelines:

Warm-up: Start with a an initial 5-10 minutes warming-up routine to help prepare your body to the demands of workouts. These could be mobility exercises as well as dynamic stretching, gentle aerobic.

Make sure you are doing the correct exercises. Pick exercises specifically targeted at the muscles of the shoulders and their the joints around them. Examples of this include shoulder press posterior raises and the rotator cuff exercises.

Utilize proper posture: Be sure that you use the proper posture during the exercise in order to avoid injury or strain. Be aware of the alignment and posture of your body as well as avoiding reaching out or stretching to far.

Gradually increase your intensity Increase intensities of your exercise over time in order to keep improving the stability of your shoulders. This is done through increasing the weight, resistance or the number of repetitions you do your exercises or by cutting down on interval between sets.

Cool down: End with a an interval of 5 to 10 minutes for a cool-down routine for your body to recuperate and get ready for your next workout. This could involve static stretches as well as foam rolling.

If you follow these guidelines that you follow, you'll be able to successfully perform exercises for shoulder stability and increase the stability of your shoulder. Be aware of your body's signals and stop exercise if you feel any pain or discomfort. It is also important to talk with a medical professional or an instructor certified in fitness before beginning any new workout routine.

Chapter 18: Upper Body Push

The upper body push exercise is workouts that entail pressing or pushing movements that utilize the muscles in the upper part of the body, including the shoulders, chest and the triceps. The exercises aim to tone and build strength in the muscles involved, and they are performed with various kinds of equipment including barbells, dumbbells or other machines.

Examples of upper body push-up exercises are:

Bench press: Bench press is an iconic upper body exercise that requires pressing a body weight upwards while lying on the bench. It targets chest muscles shoulder, triceps, as well as shoulders.

The Push-ups. Push-ups are lower body weight exercise which involves pushing the body upwards when in the plank place. They focus on the chest shoulder, triceps muscles, as well as shoulders.

Shoulder press: A shoulder press is a training exercise for the body that requires pressing upwards a weight either from a standing or seated posture. The exercise targets the shoulders and the triceps.

Dips: Dips are an upper-body push-up exercise, which involves pushing your body up from suspended positions with the help of bars or handles. The triceps are the focus as well as the chest and shoulders.

Doing upper body pushes will help strengthen and tone muscles in the upper part of your body, increase posture and decrease the chance of injuries. It is generally suggested to incorporate several upper-body push exercises into a comprehensive fitness regimen.

There are a variety of theories about the best way to perform the upper body push exercise to build and tone muscles of the upper back. Here are some of them:

Theory of Progressive Overload Based on the progressive overload concept, the ideal method to increase the strength and mass of your muscles is gradually increasing intensities of workouts throughout time. This is done through adding amount of weight, resistance or repetitions for the exercises you are doing, or cutting down on the time between sets.

Theory of Specificity: The specificity theory suggests that the most effective method to increase the strength of your muscles and increase muscle mass is to do exercises which specifically target muscles you wish to strengthen. When it comes to upper body pushes This could include activities that include bench press as well as push-ups and shoulders press.

Theory of individual differences Individual differences theory indicates that the ideal approach to build the strength and mass of muscles can differ based on the person's particular characteristics like the level of fitness, age and medical background. The theory stresses the importance of tailoring fitness plans to each person's individual desires and needs.

Theory of periodization: The theory of idea of a periodization is that the most effective method to increase muscular strength and mass include arranging your training programme into certain stages or cycles for example, the base phase, a strength phase, or maintenance phase. This could help avoid the overtraining process and help to maximize your progress.

When you consider these ideas as well as deciding on exercises and methods which are suitable to the specific needs and goals of yours it is possible to effectively do exercise for your upper body, and build strength and muscle strength in the upper part of your body.

The practice of upper body push could provide many benefits for the fascia that connective tissue which surrounds and helps support the muscles of the body. Here are some instances of ways that upper body push exercises may benefit the fascia

Increased flexibility: Upper body exercise can enhance flexibility in the fascia through expanding and stretching the connective tissue. This could help decrease stiffness in muscles and increase flexibility and range of motion.

Improved circulation: Upper body exercise can help increase the circulation of the fascia through increasing the flow of blood to muscles as well as the tissues surrounding them. It can aid in bringing nutrition and oxygen to tissues and promote healthful fascia function.

Greater strength: Upper exercise for the body can assist strengthen the fascia through placing stress and tension on connecting tissue. This will help improve the strength overall and endurance of the fascia.

Better posture: Upper-body exercise can improve posture through strengthening the fascia and muscles in the upper part of the body. It can aid in aligning the spine and shoulders in an upright position and reduce tension on the fascia and adjacent tissues.

The overall effect of performing upper-body push-ups could provide many benefits for the fascia such as improved flexibility, increased blood flow, improved strength as well as improved posture.

For upper body exercise and build and tone muscles of the upper back take these steps:

Warm-up: Start with a an initial 5-10 minutes warming-up routine to get your body ready to the demands of workouts. It could include exercises for mobility as well as dynamic stretching, moderate cardiovascular.

Pick the correct exercises Choose upper-body push-up exercises which target muscles that you'd like to strengthen. Some examples include bench presses and push-ups as well as shoulder presses and dips.

Utilize the correct form: Be sure you follow the correct form while performing exercises in order to prevent injury or strain. Take note of how you posture, and align and adhere to the precise guidelines for each exercise.

Gradually increase your intensity gradually increasing your intensity over time for continued improvement in the strength of your muscles and mass. It can be accomplished by increasing the weight or resistance, or repetitions for your exercise, or even by reducing the interval between sets.

Cool down: Follow up with a an interval of 5-10 minutes for a cool-down routine to aid your body heal and prepare for the next workout. This could involve static stretches as well as foam rolling.

If you follow these guidelines that you follow, you'll be able to successfully perform the upper body and push-up exercises to build and strengthen the muscles in the upper part of your body. Make sure to pay attention to your body, and halt if there is any discomfort or discomfort. Also, it is important to speak with a medical professional or qualified fitness trainer prior to beginning an exercise routine.

Upper Body Pull

The upper body pull exercise is exercises that incorporate the movement of pulling or rowing using the muscles in the upper part of the body, like those in the back, biceps and forearms. The exercises aim to tone and build strength in the muscles involved, and they are performed with various forms of equipment, including barbells, dumbbells and machines.

Examples of upper body pull exercises are:

Lat pull-down pull-down can be described as an upper-body pull workout which involves pulling a heavy object down from a sitting posture using a bar, or cable. It is a workout for the back muscles and, in particular the lats.

For a lat pull-down exercise to strengthen and tone those muscles in the back, perform these instructions:

Make sure to adjust the machine. Position yourself directly in close proximity to the pull-down lat machine, and alter the height of your seat so that the handles are an arm's height while you're in a seated position.

Grab the handles with your hands: grip the handles by using an overhand grip. Place your hands slightly more than shoulder width to each other.

Sit down Relax on the bench, and then tilt your back while keeping your feet on the floor, and your core active.

Keep your elbows in close proximity to your body Pull the handles downwards toward your chest. Breathe as you pull.

The arms are extended slowly. Slowly, extend your arms until you return to their starting position Inhale while doing as you do.

Repeat: Repetition the exercise until you have completed the desired number of times.

It's crucial to maintain proper posture when performing the pull-down exercises for your lats to prevent injury or strain. Keep your core firmly engaged. Avoid the swing or use of momentum and stop when you feel discomfort or pain. Also, it's a good idea to speak with a medical specialist or certified fitness instructor prior to beginning a new fitness programme.

Row: A row is a upper-body pull workout that requires pulling weights towards your body when in a seated or standing place. The exercise targets the back muscles, the biceps, as well as the forearms.

For the exercise to be performed to strengthen and tone your Biceps, back muscle and forearms, you must follow these instructions:

Select the equipment you will use This exercise could be accomplished using a variety of tools, including dumbbells, barbells, or even a machine. Pick the right equipment most suitable to your fitness level and objectives.

Set yourself up: Sit in front of the machine with your legs wide apart, with your knees bent slightly. If you are using dumbbells, keep the weights at arm's length between your legs using an overhand hold. If you're using a barbell, or machine, set yourself in accordance with the directions.

Engage your core muscles: Contract the core muscles in order to support your spine and keep your posture in good shape throughout the workout.

The Row: While keeping your elbows near towards your body. draw the weight toward your chest and squeeze the shoulder blades. Breathe as you pull.

The arms are extended slowly. Slowly, extend your arms until you return to their starting point Inhaling while doing as you do.

Repeat Repeat the exercise until you have completed the desired amount of repetitions.

It is essential to follow the correct technique when doing the exercise of rowing to prevent injury or strain. Keep your body's core in place, stay away from the swing or use of momentum and stop when you feel discomfort or pain. Also, it's a good idea to talk with a health expert or a certified fitness instructor prior to beginning a new fitness regimen.

Bicep curl: A Bicep curl is a upper body pull workout which involves curving a weight upwards toward the shoulder while in an elevated posture. The biceps are the focus of this exercise.

To do the Bicep Curl exercise to strengthen and tone your biceps adhere to these guidelines:

Pick the right equipment for you Bicep curls can be done with different equipment like dumbbells, barbell, or even a machine. Select the one that's most suitable to your fitness level and objectives.

Place yourself in front of the machine with your legs wide apart, with your knees bent slightly. If you're using dumbbells hold them in between your legs using an uninvolved grip. If you are using a barbell, or machine, place your body according to guidelines.

Engage your core muscles: Contract the core muscles in order to help stabilize your spine. This will allow you to keep your posture in good shape throughout the workout.

Curl: With your elbows near to your side, you can extend your arms, and then curl the weight to your shoulders. Breathe as you curl.

The arms are extended slowly. Slowly, extend your arms until you return to their starting position and inhale as you do as you do.

Repeat: Repetition the exercises until you reach your desired number of times.

It's crucial to maintain proper posture when you perform the bicep curl to prevent injury or strain. Keep your core engaged and avoid doing a swing or using momentum or stop if you notice any discomfort or pain. Also, it's a good idea to speak with a medical specialist or a certified fitness instructor prior to beginning a new fitness programme.

Pull-ups: A pull-up is an exercise for the upper body that requires pulling the body up from a suspended posture using either handles or a bar. The exercise targets the back muscles, the biceps, as well as the forearms.

To do the pull-up workout to strengthen and tone your Biceps, back muscle and forearms, you must follow these instructions:

Pick the right equipment for you This exercise could be accomplished using a variety of tools, including rings, bars, or handles. Select the one that's most appropriate to your fitness level and objectives.

Place yourself in front of to the machine and hold the handles or bar with an overhand grip. Place your hands slightly larger than shoulder width apart.

Engage your core muscles: Contract the core muscles in order to support your spine and keep your posture in good shape throughout the workout.

Keep your elbows near the body's, push your body up towards the handles or bar. Inhale while pulling.

Lower body Then slowly lower your body until it is back to the original place, breathing in as you go.

Repeat: Repetition the exercises until you reach your desired amount of times.

It is essential to follow the correct technique when doing the pull-up workout to avoid injury or strain. Keep your body's core in place, stay away from moving your body or swinging, or stop if you notice any discomfort or pain. It is also recommended to talk with a health expert or certified fitness trainer prior to starting any new workout regimen. If you're unable to pull yourself up in a complete manner however, you could alter the workout by using bands for support or perform negative reps (lowering your body slowly from the highest place). If you are getting more powerful, you may gradual increase the difficulty applying a tighter grip, or by adding weight.

Engaging in upper body pull exercises helps to build strength and tone muscles in the upper part of your body, enhance posture and decrease the likelihood of injury. It's recommended to incorporate several upper-body pull exercises into a comprehensive fitness programme.

Chapter 19: Accessory Elbows And Wrists

Upper body exercises are workouts that work on small muscles in the upper part of the body, including the elbow as well as wrist extensors as well as flexors. They are frequently employed to enhance a complete training program, and are able increase endurance, strength, and stability performance in these regions.

Here are some examples of exercises for upper body which target elbows and wrists:

Wrist curl: A wrist curl is an exercise which requires flexing and stretching the wrist with the aid of a weight. It is performed sitting or standing, and is completed using a dumbbell, or barbell.

Extension of wrists: A wrist extension exercise requires extending your wrist with the help of a weight. The exercise can be done seated or standing. It can be performed using a dumbbell or barbell.

Tricep extension: A extension of the tricep is an exercise in which you extend your elbow by using a heavy weight. It is performed sitting or standing, and is accomplished using a dumbbell cable machine, or barbell.

Bicep curl: A Bicep curl is an exercise where you bend your elbow by using an object of weight. The exercise can be done in a sitting position or standing, and could be accomplished with a barbell, dumbbell or cable machine.

If you include exercise for the upper part of your body in your routine to increase strength and stabilize the wrist joint and elbow and wrist joints, which will help lower the chance of injuries and increase the functionality of the joints. In general, it is recommended to complete these exercises with less weight as well as higher repetitions, to avoid stressing joints.

There are a variety of exercises to help increase the flexibility and strength of your wrists and elbows. Below are some examples:

Wrist curls: Lie in a seat with your feet flat and place a dumbbell into the other hand, with your palm facing upwards. Then slowly curl your wrist toward your body. Then return to a lower position. Repeat with the opposite hand.

Wrist extensions: Lie in a seat with your feet flat on the floor and place a dumbbell into the other hand, with your palm facing downwards. Then slowly raise your wrist off your body, and then lower it to return. Repeat with the opposite hand.

Forearm curls: Lie down with your arms by your sides with you have a dumbbell on each of your hands. Keep your elbows in close proximity to your body, gradually move your wrists upwards towards your chest. Then, return to a lower position.

Tricep dips: Put your hands on the seat or bench behind you, with your hands facing toward your body. Reduce yourself to a point where your elbows have been bent 90 degrees. Then, push upwards.

Stretches for elbow mobility there are a variety of stretching exercises that help increase the flexibility of your elbows. An example of this is the elbow flexion stretch that involves putting your hand straight ahead of you while gently bent your elbow in order to draw the hand toward your shoulder. The other is the elbow extension stretch. It requires you to hold your arms straight towards the side, and then gradually extending your elbow so that you draw your hand back into the body.

Through performing these and similar exercises on a regular basis, you'll increase the strength and flexibility of your wrists and elbows as well as reduce the likelihood of injuries. Make sure you start slow and slowly intensify and lengthen the duration of your exercises to build up your strength.

Chapter 20: Benefits Of Using Foam Roller

Foam rolling provides additional benefits that few know about. It is more than just relaxing sore and tired muscles (though that is certainly one of the main benefits) with a host of additional health benefits for the body, it may surprise you. In this article, we'll briefly discuss some benefits that you can get through a regular foam rolling routine. It's really hard (if but not difficult) to write down all the benefits that you are likely to receive, because there are literally numerous benefits that are too numerous to list. In addition, there are numerous benefits to foam rolling that a number of book could be written around solely the benefits of foam rolling However, scientists and health professionals discover new advantages almost every single day.

After you've read this section, you'll be able to understand the reason how foam rolling can be one of the most beneficial exercises you can perform for your body. It will be clear that rolling is an effective method of keeping well, improving your quality of life significantly, as well as avoiding numerous negative consequences that are associated with ageing. The results will show that rolling is perhaps one of the most significant and life-changing decision you've made in your life.

1. Increased Mobility

One of the consequences of ageing is an increase in mobility. In other words, tasks that were previously effortless and painless become challenging as we get older. It is possible that standing, walking and bending can be strenuous or (for certain) may be almost impossible. A lot of people believe that it's a natural process that aging goes through and that there's something we can do to prevent it. There are even physicians tell patients that the decreased mobility is just the result of "getting older" and it is normal to age.

The majority of physical therapists, particularly those who are specialized in geriatric treatment, will admit that the primary reason for limited mobility among older people is the degeneration of muscles and joint inflammation along with massive myofascial adhesions all over the body. In this chapter, one principal advantages from foam rolling is an increasing blood flow through the whole body. The elderly and the older could have poor circulation that can cause joints and ligaments to become stiff due to poor lubrication or an insufficient supply of nutrients-rich blood.

The best part is that foam rolling doesn't have to be restricted to healthy young energetic people. In fact, anybody, from three years old (perhaps older) until around 90 (perhaps or even later) is able to profit of foam rolling.

It's a particularly valuable supplement to rehabilitation programs as it is able to be applied with as little or forcefully as is needed to relax adhesions, and to enhance circulation throughout your body.

2. Pain Therapy

One of the primary advantages of foam rolling is helping ease pain from sore and exhausted muscles. However, the therapeutic benefits of foam rolling is far more than this. In addition to being very beneficial to muscles and joint therapy and rehabilitation, it is also able to aid in easing or eliminating discomforts that are often left untreated for a long time, or even treated with medication that just mask the symptoms but do not actually address the cause.

In the beginning, your muscles ligaments, joints and tendons are always being pulled, stretched and typically mistreated by means that eventually degrade them and lead to the body to "malfunction." Arthritis, tendonitis, bursitis as well as a myriad of different conditions are the result of abuse and neglect of muscles over a long time, which can cause discomfort in the later years and often hindering mobility. Through the use of the right techniques for foam rolling (which will be discussed later in this book) to stop these diseases or even treat them.

An everyday routine of foam rolling particularly for the back of your upper and shoulders, may provide an extremely deep and relaxing release for these nerves. It does this in easing the muscles and tissues and providing to maintain a healthy balance in your head and neck. Numerous people have commented over how well foam rolling helped ease their headaches. However, headaches aren't the only discomforts and aches that foam rolling can ease.

3. Improved Functions Of Our Vital Organs

It's not just that increasing blood flow (by breaking down fascial adhesions) reduce and in many cases relieve suffering, but also our organs are able to function in peak efficiency, performing their work at the level they perform most efficient. It's not necessary to remind that it's vital for your heart to continue to circulate blood through the body. Or how crucial it is for your kidneys to be able to remove waste out of your blood, and to regulate the levels of water in your body.

Through the release of fascial adhesions with foam rolling, you can increase blood flow and ensure that your vital organs receive the right quantity of oxygen and nutrients to continue functioning. Numerous people have shared with me that they hoped to feel that mobility will improve and that tension and discomforts might be eased however, they were pleasantly shocked (and frequently amazed) at how much better they felt all over after adhering to a regular routine. The benefits from foam rolling that are directly linked to improving the health the function of organs vital to us.

4. Improved Vitality

If your organs are receiving the right circulation of blood, your health levels naturally improve because your body is getting back to working as it was designed to. Healthy circulation is essential for our general well-being and health.

One of the things that I've received from one of those who have chosen to try foam rolling, and who have adhered to a routine for about a week has been that they were pleasantly surprised at how energetic they've been. A lot of people have said they've experienced sleeping more comfortably, frequently sleeping shorter hours and feeling like they are more rested than prior to.

What's great with this level of health is that you are able to use it to push your body in more form. It is now possible to have the drive (and desire) to work out regularly to increase your fitness and endurance. It is possible that walking can be easier than ever however, it's also more fun. The blood oxygen levels will rise even higher through actions you've put off, and once the process continues, your energy levels is likely to increase. So, in essence you'll find that just starting a routine exercise routine can dramatically improve the quality of life you enjoy to levels you can't think of.

5. Reduction Of Cellulite

In case you're not familiar the term, it refers to a condition which causes skin to appear as if it has areas of sub-surface fat deposits. This creates looks lumpy and dimpled. The most common spots for it are in the abdomen, thighs and buttocks. There are numerous medical terms to describe cellulite. Some of them are dermopanniculosis, adiposis tosa, deformans or status protrususcutis. It is not necessary to be familiar with the terms used in medical literature to identify cellulite. It is commonly referred to as the orange peel syndrome, or cottage cheese's skin (which is more descriptive than medical terminology).

Although you can pay $100 for a magic cream that could (or may not) assist you in decreasing the size of your pores, but probably leave the area worse than before You will discover that foam rolling can do the trick very well and not just will it to reduce (or entirely erase) the appearance of cellulite however, it keeps the cellulite off for so long as you continue rolling.

Foam rolling is proven to help massage these areas and assist in breaking down the fat fibers interwoven that could contribute to the growth of cellulite up. The process also improves blood flow (and oxygen) to these areas, which helps keep the fibers that are underneath healthy and in good working order and also aids in helping the body eliminate waste and toxins. If you're like the thousands of other people with cellulite around your abdomen, thighs or buttocks within just a couple of weeks after foam rolling, you'll observe that your cellulite appears to melt away with no extra supplements or dangerous creams.

Foam rolling is beneficial to us because it helping us break down numerous adhesions, which cause the body to fight to provide oxygen and nutrients to the organs. A variety of grave conditions are due to poor circulation.

Our circulation is not only increased and our organs are receiving the nutrients and oxygen they require, but also the muscles, tendons and joints also improve and our mobility is increased and allowing us to participate in more enjoyable activities that we are able to take part in.

I could go on for days about the many benefits I've learned from customers and acquaintances who have tried the foam roller a go and I'm convinced that the best method to grasp the benefits of foam rolling is to try the benefits for yourself. Foam rollers cost nothing they can be stored conveniently and they are a lot of fun to operate when you are able to master the use of it.

So, foam rolling while needing a commitment to do it daily, is a fun activity that you'll find enjoyable, and looking at it every day.

Chapter 21: Different Types Of Massage Rollers

foam rolling is a method to effectively to strengthen a variety of muscles, including TFL trapezius, hip flexors, rhomboids quadriceps, hamstrings and piriformis. It also helps to strengthen the latissimus for and gastrocnemius. Through rolling the muscles on the foam roller, and maintaining a certain level of pressure, these muscles areas can relax and be relaxed. It's time to look at the tools used to perform this technique of self-massage.

It is an excellent option to warm up or for recovering. In your practice to warm up Foam rolling can prepare your body for the strenuous exercise you'll need to perform. It can improve blood circulation. When blood is properly circulated is reduces the chance of suffering injuries. After an exercise foam rolling is highly suggested. It could help speed up the recuperation time as it also increases blood flow to your muscles and can help bring in vital nutrients and oxygen to the muscles.

The foam roller usually comes made of an oblong. There are a variety of dimensions, however the one most frequently used size is approximately 6 inches in diameter, and around 12 inches in length. Long foam rollers nevertheless, are at least 36 inches in length. These are usually employed for back use. As you're a novice to the art of foam rolling, it's best to begin by using the gentle variety. For you to get familiar but, I'll introduce you to the various sizes and shapes of foam rolling.

In the first place be aware that there are two primary varieties of foam rollers.

1. The foam roller EVA

2. The EVE high-density foam roll.

EVA rollers are particularly comfortable. It is advantageous if you're looking for an incredibly soft feel. Also, it could be useful to you when you are a novice. Its downside is that it can flatten quickly. It's a blessing if you're able to create EVA foam rollers last for for a year.

Its EVE foam roller however provides a more firm feeling. Although it's not as gentle like EVA rollers, however EVE's are able to stand up to the rigors of use. They are able to last for many years.

How can you tell them different? A roller can be identified through the colour. EVA rollers are typically white, while high-density EVE rollers are usually darker shades. The majority of them are black. Additionally, EVA rollers have a silky surface. EVE rollers, on contrary, are much more rough. They could look as if there are tiny pellets sitting in the middle.

You must be on guard! Make sure you are aware.

1. Soft Body Roller

The type of roller suggested to beginners, however non-beginners may are also able to use the foam roller. The body soft roller is perfect for people who like gentle contact. It is possible to massage the major muscles with this soft rolling device. It is perfect for legs and back.

For beginners, they start using foam rollers bigger in diameter. If the area of the foam roller is greater, then rolling can be more comfortable. This is because the force is dispersed instead of concentrated. If you're ready raise the intensity then you are able to switch to the less radial type.

2. Rumble Roller

This one is only for those who want to feel a strong touch. If you'd like to feel further, this roller is the one for those of you. But, if you're threshold for pain is not high it is best to stay away of this one.

The foam roller comes with bumps. These bumps can help let loose knots that are extremely tough. Be careful not to use this tool over a long period of time in a particular area unless do not want to injure yourself further and do more harm to the muscles.

3. Textured Foam Roller

It's a general-purpose foam roller that can be used for any purpose. If you feel that the soft roller is too soft however the hard roller isn't enough for your needs. This will provide you with an extra amount of intensity. It will give you a bit greater pressure from this.

The foam roller has been constructed with grooves and bumps. This type of design lets users to focus on the tight spots. The roller can be moved around on the areas that are tight. When using the foam roller with textured surfaces but, it is possible to stop at that particular area. You can work on relaxing and contracting the muscles as you lay in the rolling. The bumps and grooves will perform the job for you.

4. Cold Foam Roller

If you're looking for some relief from the heat that isn't too heavy, this might be the ideal roller to choose. It is a great option to ease aching injuries or pains.

Cold foam is constructed out of stainless steel. If you're feeling achy following your exercise, you can roll the cold ball on your muscles and joints that have been sore. It will provide immediate relief which is better than the traditional cold bath. Cold foam rollers offer more rapid healing time as well as a lower chance of swelling.

5. Textured Ball Roller

You don't want to feel extreme pressure, however you have some sore places that you have to treat. The foam roller is the right tool for people like you.

The balls in this roller are able to be targeted at small muscle groups, including the hips. This is a great option for concentrated stress. In reality you are able to alter the firmness of the roll in accordance with how tight your muscles feel. The best way to do this is to make adjustments by using a needle inflation pump.

6. Foot Roller

This product is great for people with fatigued feet, particularly the feet of runners. The special roller was designed to ease tight soles. Put it on your calves or on your feet. The foot roller is utilized for smaller areas. It's constructed of strong knobs that resemble the fingers of a massage professional.

Do not apply pressure directly to your most tight muscle. This won't work as well as you'd hope it would be. This is because the muscle that is tightest is likely to be strained. This makes it much more difficult to allow it to ease up. If your muscle isn't at ease when you massage it and massage it, it will not result in any kind of result.

It is possible to focus on strengthening the lower limbs first. Begin by rolling down until you reach your feet. Start with rolling your hips and back using an lacrosse ball. Then, you can shift the ball towards the torso prior to starting rolling your feet from the legs down to your feet.

7. Adjustable Foam Roller

The adjustable roller can be described as the ultimate knot buster. It was specifically designed to eliminate knots and kinks in your hamstrings, calves, and quads.

Instead of placing your body upon the roller, grip the ergonomic handles on the roller and move it to your desired area. Simply press the bar into the area with both directions. The curved roller will make sure that your muscle is being treated correctly.

The disks that make up this roller are able to rotate while you press both up and down in order to unwind knots. The handle is yours to control so you are able to press as lightly or forcefully as you want.

If you feel it is too painful it is causing pain in your spot Try taking deep breaths. This can ease the discomfort.

8. Wand Foam Roller

The runners will benefit the most from this foam wand. It is a variant of the roller that is adjustable and has a handles. This wand features the help of a piece of foam. It can be gently rolled across your IT band the quads, hamstrings, and calves. Don't rush through the procedure. You should roll as slowly as you are able to so that your fascia is able to relax. The efficiency of your session of rolling is contingent on this.

Chapter 22: Foam Rolling Safety Tips

Foam rolling was once an exclusive activity for professionals, coaches, as well as physical therapy professionals. Now, it is routine. Due to its advantages for fitness, it is widely practiced by people of all degrees of fitness.

The majority of them began in the same place you're at, unsure and unclear. In order to help you through this process I've set out below some of the basics for you to follow when rolling foam. Make sure you adhere to them, and you will surely enjoy the many advantages of this technique of self-myofascial release.

1. First, stretch. You should be excited to begin. Before stretching, do a stretch the muscle that you'll be working on the first. Stretch before rolling over that particular muscle. The stretch doesn't have to be a complicated one in the event that it's correctly heated up.

2. Place your body in a proper position. The foam roller must be placed under your body. Your body should be directly on the roller.

3. Be prepared for discomfort. As we said before, a bit of discomfort or pain is to be to be expected. If you're working on an area of trigger, the discomfort could radiate to different areas of your body, too. This is common.

4. Use gentle pressure- It is important to apply your body's weight to the area you want to exert pressure. Begin slowly, and end at a level that you are able to bear. Move the target between each other.

5. Do not stop until the pain is gone. The main concern is to target tight spots. They can be particularly sensitive. You should also work on the areas with inflexibility. Foam rolling helps regulate the blood flow. The process will not only help to solve knots.

Additionally, it will help increase the flexibility of muscles.

6. Avoid rolling on bones and joints. Roll on soft tissues and muscles. Do not roll directly on your bones and joints. Foam rolling will do nothing on these tough parts besides in the case of pain.

7. Be careful not to roll too fastto properly exercise muscles, it is important to slow down your roll. Fast rolling in a back-andforth movement isn't recommended. It is best to not exceed one inch per second.

The speed of your roll may be more beneficial, but in order to effectively treat knots, you must use slow and controlled movements. That is how you will get to the goal, that is to loosen muscles and loosen the fascia. It is not possible to release the fascia quickly. The fascia is comprised of the fibrous, thick and dense web of tissues. Doing it in one go will not do the trick.

8. Avoid staying at the same place for an extended period of time. foam rolling isn't an endurance test. It's not a matter of how long you're able to handle it. If you are prone to rubbing one area over a long period of time can cause more harm. There is a chance of hurting or damaging tissue, or even irritating the nerve. It could result in bruises. It could, in reality cause inflammation, which is what you do not would.

9. Avoid rolling directly onto the affected area- If the affected area is painful even to roll the area, it may be a sign of that it is a single issue. The region is damaged. Do not roll on it constantly because it could create more stress and can make inflammation even more severe. Concentrate on the connective tissue. Apply the tension gradually.

10. Be aware of your posture and formfor the best results from foam rolling, it is essential to adhere to the right posture and

correct manner of doing things. If you don't, you could cause more harm than good. If you feel exhausted to roll, then take the time to relax. It's important to ensure that you remain concentrated throughout the whole exercise.

11. Don't roll your lower back. It's okay to roll your upper back however, it's best to stay clear of foam rolling your lower back. The use of a foam roller on this part of the body will make the spine contract in an attempt to prevent. If you're suffering from problems with the back of your lower it is possible to use tennis or lacrosse balls instead. Better yet, talk to an expert on the most effective solution to this problems.

12. You should wait 1 to two days prior to another sessionIt's not recommended to do foam rolling every two days. While you should perform this routinely however, you must rest for 24 or 48 hours before your next session. While you wait, keep hydrated. Be aware that trigger points can

be caused by aspects of your life, including diet. Implement healthy changes to your eating habits. You must be refreshed.

13. Talk to your physician first.and then try foam rolling. It can be very helpful. However, it shouldn't be advised for everyone. people suffering from skin disorders or bleeding issues, kidney disease heart, organ problems should steer clear using this procedure unless the physician has approved the procedure for them. Make sure to consult your physician. Health professionals can provide additional advice regarding the proper usage of the method so you get the most benefit from it.

Remember these rules to keep in mind while doing foam rolling exercises.

Chapter 23: The Exercises

1. Inner Thigh (Adductor)

The inner thigh foam roller is the ideal exercise for thighs that are tight, as it will expand them. Yu certainly will enjoy this exercise that uses foam rollers to provide give a full massage. If you apply the circular foam roller across your lower thigh area and thighs, you can loosen up the tough connective tissue, and reduce muscle stiffness.

How to Do Inner Thigh Foam Rolling

Place yourself in an incline stance, balancing using your elbows and toes.

Spread your entire round foam roller on 45 degrees to the body.

You can gently open your left knee, as you rotate your foot around your hip.

Place your left side on the entire round foam roller that is jus above your knee.

Roll the roller slowly starting from your knee and moving towards the inner thigh.

Try to keep as much of weight you are able to.

Repeat the entire procedure using the other leg.

2. Biceps Release

Muscles in the body are known to perform in pairs. Well it is when the biceps form the dominant overs, they contract, bending the arm. In contrast the triceps will respond with they release. As the triceps contract the biceps relax, and your arm is able to straighten out. Be aware that if one muscle group is not balanced against the opposite muscle group, tension can rise. It is therefore essential to roll foam for biceps relaxation.

How to Do Foam Rolling For Biceps Release

Lay down lying down facing downwards with your left arm extended towards the side with your left arm placed in a position that is comfortable in order to provide the necessary support.

Position the complete round foam roller on the top of your left Biceps.

Press gently into the roller of foam.

Keep your hand in to the position you are in for a couple of minutes.

Move your body slowly and move the foam roller around your biceps.

Use static force to get rid of any tight spots and keep it in place until you can.

Be sure that you breathe deeply and slowly.

Repeat the whole procedure to the other arm.

3. Total Calf Release

In all muscle groups within the human body the calves are among the ones most affected by genes. They are, in general, the toughest muscles to develop. But, it is possible to enhance the condition and size that your calves. One of the unique characteristics that calves possess is the fact that they are able to exercise more regularly than the other muscles. The ideal exercise to maintain well-maintained calves is complete calves' release.

How to Do Total Calf Release Foam Rolling

Place your feet on the ground while your legs straighten out and the hands are positioned behind you lifting the weight.

Place a complete round foam roller between your knees.

You can slowly roll down your back legs, side-by-side between your knees until your ankles.

Continue to roll until you reach an area that is tender, the apply pressure to it.

4. Hamstring Release

Hamstring release is a great exercise to decrease hyper-tonicity of the hamstring. The exercise follows the standard of counter-strain in order to correct problems between antagonist and agonist muscles. The goal behind hamstring release can include but not be only about improving posture and balance in sitting as well as limiting internal rotation during the gait cycle; increasing the length of stride; reducing excessive pull, which can lead to hip dislocations; reducing the ankle's compensatory force; and eliminating the ineffective crouched gait pattern.

How to Do Hamstring Release

Sit in your left foot on a oval foam roller.

Flex your left knee and put your hands to support you.

Then, roll back and forth starting from your knee until just below your right cheek.

Change legs, then continue the entire exercise.

5. Lower Back (Erector Spinae)

Foam rolling along the lower back can help extend the abdominal and lower back muscles. This exercise will also train your pelvis in a neuromuscular way when you shift from one place to the next. The purpose of this workout is to focus on mid back movements. This particular exercise isn't suitable for those who are injured or weak back and lumbar spine.

How to Do Foam Rolling for Lower Back

Lay on the ground with your back facing upwards, then put a complete circular foam roller over your back. Place it just under the shoulder blades.

Place your hands on your neck to provide assistance.

Arch your back across the foam roller and keep your legs and hips onto the mat.

Stay in the same location for several minutes, then relax and continue the stretch for several repetitions.

6. Piriformis (Upper Buttocks)

Piriformis is located within the gluteal region which assists in rotating the thigh's exterior. The Piriformis are an extremely important muscle group that is mobile and can improve stability. This exercise is simple to perform and the outcomes can be extremely beneficial for overall health of the body and its mobility.

How to Foam Roll for Piriformis

Begin in a sitting in a full-circle foam roller with your right leg is crossed over the left knee.

Utilize your right hand to help support your weight by placing it down to the side behind your back.

The foam roller over the outer of your hips, just below the gluteal zone.

Change legs and the supporting place and repeat the exercise.

7. Glute Massage

Glute Massage with foam rollers release glutes that are locked by sitting. Glute release effectively improves blood flow to hip muscles and decreases the back strain caused by glutes, as well as it can help to loosen hips as and the lower back. It is recommended to stay clear of this workout when you feel a sharp pain or suffering from acute sciatica. Additionally, it is important to remain within a narrow range of motion in case you've undergone an operation to replace your hip.

How to Do Glute Massage

You can gently place yourself in a comfortable position on the floor. the full-round foam roller below your feet.

Chapter 24: Lacrosse Ball And Spiky Ball Workouts

Lacrosse Ball Exercises

1. Glutes Massage

Stand back against a wall and the ball from lacrosse.

You can sway from side to side and then up as well down to locate an area of softness.

Let the ball press down on the area Relax your body weight against the wall.

Once your pain is gone keep this position for 30 minutes.

Repeat on the opposite side.

2. Hamstrings Massage

You should sit on a firm chair that is sufficient high off the ground so that your legs can sit.

Place the ball under your thigh then move it around until you can find a comfortable place.

Then slowly bend and extend your knee for 30 seconds.

3. Upper Shoulders And Back

Using a soccer ball between your back and wall, put your back against the wall.

Place the ball onto the spine on one side.

Make a move in all directions until you locate the soft spot.

4. Foot Massage

If you put your feet placed on the floor, relax your feet.

Below the arch of your foot, place the ball of lacrosse.

Slowly roll the ball through the arch of your foot.

Common Spiky Ball Exercises

1. Shoulder Release

Stand on your Spiky Ball against the wall

By applying pressure to the regions that are tight, use your weight with your body to push the ball.

2. Gluteal Release

Lay on your back with your feet flat on ground with your knees bent.

Slip Your Spiky Ball underneath your buttocks.

Smoothly move your ball till you locate the trigger point.

To raise the pressure, allow the knee that is on the injured side extend towards the other side.

3. Foot Release

Put it under your foot. Spiky Ball underneath your foot.

Use your body weight onto the foot and push the ball off the heel toward your toes.